Anti-Inflammatory
Eating Made Easy

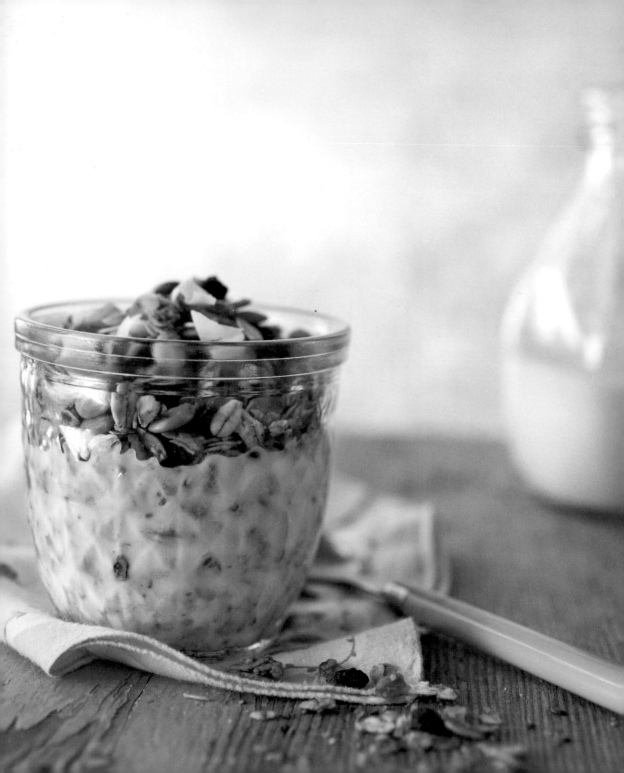

Anti-Inflammatory
Eating Made Easy

—»»——⸻«««—

NUTRITION PLAN and 75 RECIPES
for a HEALTHIER BODY

—»»——⸻«««—

MICHELLE BABB, MS, RD, CD
Photography by Hilary McMullen

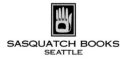

SASQUATCH BOOKS
SEATTLE

To my husband, who is my number one recipe tester, and my mom, who is my biggest cheerleader

Printed in China

Published by Sasquatch Books

19 18 17   9 8 7 6 5

Editor: Gary Luke
Project editor: Em Gale
Design: Anna Goldstein
Photography: Hilary McMullen
Food styling: Julie Hopper
Copy editor: Rachelle Longé McGhee

Library of Congress Cataloging-in-Publication Data is available.

ISBN: 978-1-57061-933-5

Sasquatch Books
1904 Third Avenue, Suite 710
Seattle, WA 98101
(206) 467-4300
www.sasquatchbooks.com
custserv@sasquatchbooks.com

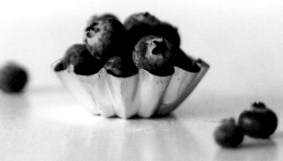

Table of Contents

Recipe List

BREAKFASTS

HEALTHY SNACKS

SOUPS AND STEWS

SALADS AND SIDES

VEGETARIAN MAIN DISHES

PESCATARIAN MAIN DISHES

Hazelnut-Encrusted Halibut with Dipping Sauce	137
Poached White Fish with Mango Lime Chutney	139
Pan-Fried Sardines with Sautéed Kale and Chard	141
Salmon en Papillote with Silky Celery Root Puree	142
Mediterranean Salmon Skewers	144
Pumpkin Coconut Curry with White Fish	146
Sizzling Salmon and Quinoa Skillet	147
Nori-Wrapped Mackerel with Wasabi "Mayo"	149
Fish Taco Salad with Strawberry Avocado Salsa	151
Oven-Roasted Black Cod with Smashed Sweet Peas	153

HINT-OF-MEAT MAIN DISHES

Moroccan Lamb Tagine with Chickpeas and Apricots	159
Bison Lettuce Cups with Garnet Yam Home Fries	160
Spring Lamb Stew	163
Steak Salad with Massaged Kale	164
Veggie Beef Burger with Rocket Salad	166
Sweet Potato Shepherd's Pie	168

DESSERTS

Pumpkin Coconut Pie with Almond Crust	173
Mixed Berry Walnut Crumble	177
Rustic Pear and Fig Crostatas	178
So-Easy Coconut Mango Sorbet	180
Baked Pears or Apples with Cashew Cream	182
Strawberry Rhubarb Crumble	183
Vanilla Wafer Pudding	185
No-Bake Peach Pie	186

Foreword

If you are lucky enough to be a friend of Michelle's, she has fed you delicious meals. If you are lucky enough to be her client, she has taught you how to feed yourself well. I am lucky enough to be both a friend and colleague. We've eaten many meals together, have co-taught anti-inflammatory classes, and have shared hundreds of patients. Why do I send my patients to Michelle? Because she gets them better, and her tools are simple: real food. It's a prescription that I write often: "Michelle Babb, RD, Anti-Inflammatory Diet." We have observed over the years that our patients who adopt a Mediterranean-style anti-inflammatory diet feel better. We note tremendous improvements in joint pain, inflammation, cardiovascular disease, and weight. We encourage our shared patients to eat this way because it is sustainable, delicious, celebrates seasonal food, and is supported by research showing that this is the way we should all be eating.

We know it can be intimidating to change what you eat. If you are concerned that switching to an anti-inflammatory diet means a sacrifice of sorts, you will be thrilled to try out the recipes in this book! Embrace them fully and serve them to dinner guests and your family. Take Michelle's Creamy Avocado Spinach Dip (page 66) to your next gathering, and I guarantee you will be asked for the recipe. Serve Mediterranean Salmon Skewers (page 144) and Warm Brussels Sprout Salad with Pecans and Currants (page 101) to your family and see that we all love eating this way.

Michelle and I are part of a revolution of getting people back to eating real, whole foods. This book will not only give you the tools to heal your body but will also expand your palate and introduce you to new ingredients, flavors, and cooking techniques that aren't difficult. I'm thrilled to see Michelle weave together in one book her knowledge of nutrition and mindful eating, her years of feeding her friends and family, and her insights into what people are looking for when they ask, "What can I eat?"

—*Dr. Katherine Oldfield, naturopathic physician and owner of the*
West Seattle Natural Medicine Clinic

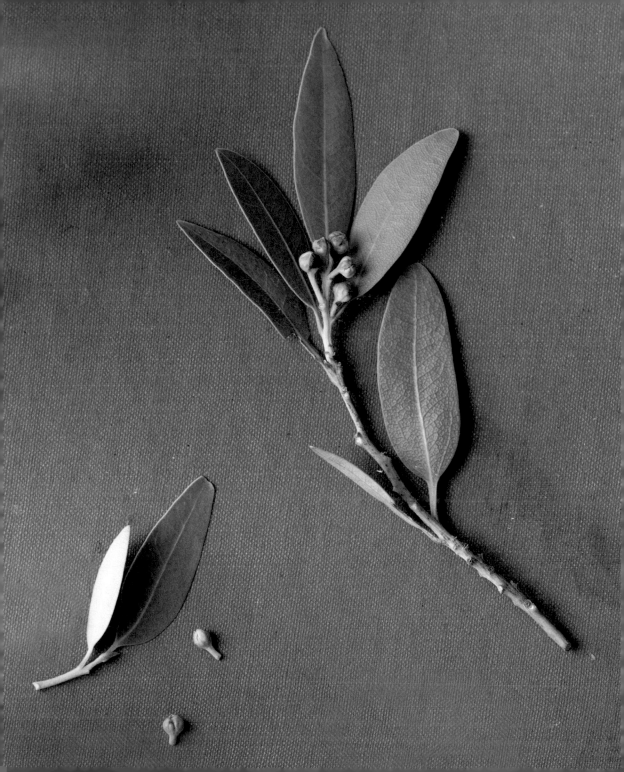

Introduction

Inflammation has become the latest buzzword in health and wellness circles, and it's making a name for itself as the underlying cause of a plethora of diseases. Having been in the nutrition field for over seventeen years, I've seen a lot of fad diets come and go, so I'm never too quick to jump on the latest diet bandwagon. What I find compelling about anti-inflammatory eating is that it's grounded in science and it's proven itself effective over, and over, and over again. That's because it's based on a Mediterranean-style diet. We can look back through decades of research and hundreds of studies that confirm that a Mediterranean diet, rich in plant-based foods and healthy fats and oils, helps reduce the risk of diabetes, cardiovascular disease, and cancer.

Every day in my private practice I see patients who are suffering from chronic conditions that are rooted in inflammation. Sometimes it manifests in obvious ways, like joint pain and general achiness in the body; other times it shows up as digestive distress, weight gain, or skin issues. Whatever the case may be, food can be a potent remedy to cool down the inflammation and restore balance in the body.

As a holistic-minded nutritionist, I'm always interested in helping patients uncover the underlying cause of chronic dysfunction. I consider it my role to empower people to use diet, exercise, sleep, stress management, and attitude to heal themselves. Making lifestyle changes isn't always easy for people, but when they start to feel the undeniable transformations, it becomes its own motivation. Even making relatively small changes to the diet can start to produce significant results.

Weight loss is frequently one of those results that make it easier for people to want to continue following an anti-inflammatory eating plan. My clients who are feeling stuck at an undesirable weight are often surprised to learn that when the body is in a state of chronic inflammation, it's often difficult to lose weight. Not to mention that carrying extra fat actually produces more inflammation.

So instead of using calorie-restrictive diets, I simply guide my clients toward the types of foods that help them deal with inflammation and, low and behold, they begin to shed the pounds.

All of the recipes in this book contain wholesome ingredients that play a key role in reversing the body's inflammatory processes. I use evidence-based nutrition to make decisions about which foods to incorporate or omit, but I don't need to bore you with the details (although I couldn't resist weaving in a few nuggets for your intellectual enjoyment!). Just know that while the combination of ingredients may be therapeutic, the goal was to create delicious and simple recipes that can be enjoyed by anyone.

I've included information about the 21-day nutritional cleanse that I use with my clients to help them reduce inflammation and restore balance in their bodies. If you're suffering from chronic inflammation or you're drawn to the idea of a "detox" or a "cleanse," this is a very safe and effective protocol that includes plenty of nutrient-rich foods and a good balance of protein, fat, and carbs. All of the recipes in this book are suitable for someone on the cleanse as well as anyone who is on an elimination diet or has multiple food allergies. Doing the cleanse is absolutely optional. Simply eating more of the foods featured in this book would be enough to put you on the path toward a healthier, more anti-inflammatory lifestyle.

You'll find a number of useful tools in this book including sample menu plans, shopping lists, guidelines for essential pantry items, and seventy-five recipes to support your health and wellness goals. If you allow yourself to embrace the concepts in this book, you'll quickly discover that this is not just another diet, but rather a way of life. May you learn to nourish yourself well, savor every delicious morsel, and feel the joy of restoring balance in your body.

Recognizing and Reducing Inflammation

Inflammation is your body's way of responding to injury and insults. It's a natural and healthy response when your body is in a state of alarm, and it helps aid in the healing process. For example, if you stumbled and twisted your ankle, you would probably experience all of the hallmarks of inflammation (swelling, redness, heat, and some loss of function). That's your body's clever way of sounding the alarm, recruiting the repair and restoration team, and preventing you from doing more harm. The important part about this kind of inflammatory response is that it has a beginning (time of injury) and an end (injury is healed).

It's the lack of an endpoint that turns this natural, healthy process into one that is dysfunctional. When the body loses its regulatory control and continues to sound the alarm bell indefinitely, the repair and restoration team becomes overzealous. It would be like using a fire hose to water the delicate plants in your garden. Sure, the plants get water, but they're uprooted and destroyed in the process.

This type of prolonged, maladaptive inflammation is a common thread in many disease states, including:

» Allergies

» Arthritis

» Asthma

» Autoimmune conditions

» Cancer

» Cardiovascular disease

» Depression

» Digestive disorders

» Eczema

» Metabolic syndrome (prediabetes)

» Neurodegenerative diseases

» Obesity

» Psoriasis

Anti-inflammatory medications are often prescribed, but they can cause unpleasant side effects and don't address the underlying cause of the symptoms that are related to inflammation, which is why an anti-inflammatory diet can be a great place to start. What follows are some other common questions about inflammation.

How Does Inflammation Become Chronic?

Genetics can certainly play a role in chronic inflammation. People who have a family history of inflammatory conditions, such as rheumatoid arthritis or cardiovascular disease, may be predisposed to chronic inflammation. However, while genetics may be what loads the gun, it's really diet and lifestyle habits that pull the trigger. Someone with a family history of cardiovascular disease who follows a Mediterranean-style diet, exercises regularly, and does not smoke may never stoke that inflammatory flame.

Even without a genetic predisposition, it's possible to create an environment of chronic inflammation in the body. This can happen for a number of reasons, including:

» Pro-inflammatory dietary choices
   » Reliance on processed foods and refined carbohydrates
   » Excess sugar
   » Too much meat, pork, poultry, eggs, and dairy
   » Not enough anti-inflammatory foods, like fish, vegetables, avocados, olives, nuts, seeds, and legumes
» Elevated stress
» Smoking
» Physical activity extremes
   » Lack of some regular form of exercise
   » Over exercising to the point of injury or not giving the body adequate recovery time between sessions

» An undiagnosed condition that's causing chronic inflammation (such as food allergies, irritable bowel syndrome, or an autoimmune disorder)

What Are the Symptoms of Chronic Inflammation?

The most obvious symptom associated with inflammation is joint pain, but there are many other ways in which inflammation can manifest in the body. For example, when clients complain of ongoing digestive problems accompanied by abdominal pain, bloating, and bowel irregularity, I know that there is inflammation in the gut. Skin issues like eczema and psoriasis are other ways in which inflammation shows up more overtly.

Some forms of inflammation are much less obvious and may go unnoticed altogether. For example, being overweight or obese puts the body in an inflammatory state because fat cells actually send out chemical messages that increase inflammation. Having high cholesterol and/or high blood sugar also initiates inflammatory processes in the body. It's really the combination of high cholesterol *with* inflammation that significantly increases the risk for heart disease.

Is There a Way to Be Tested for Inflammation?

The most common lab test for inflammation is a blood test for C-reactive protein, which is produced in the liver in response to inflammation. Practitioners may also measure sedimentation rate, which is the rate at which your red blood cells settle to the bottom of a test tube over a given time period. If there are inflammatory proteins present, the blood becomes sticky and takes more time to settle.

What Is an Anti-Inflammatory Diet?

An anti-inflammatory diet is based on a Mediterranean-style eating plan that includes plenty of vegetables, fruit, legumes, nuts, seeds, healthy oils, and fish. This may also be known as a *pescatarian diet*, because the main source of animal protein is fish and the majority of the diet is made up of plant-based foods.

There are a lot of reasons why this way of eating keeps inflammation at bay, but the most notable (and well researched) superstars in a pescatarian diet are:

OMEGA-3 FATTY ACIDS: Found mostly in seafood but also in smaller amounts in walnuts, flaxseeds, and some leafy greens like kale, omega-3s are a group of unsaturated fats that protect the body in various ways from inflammation.

FIBER: Found in plant-based foods like fruit, vegetables, whole grains, and legumes, fiber is the indigestible portion of these foods, and it's important for healthy digestion, blood sugar balance, and cholesterol management. Studies confirm a relationship between high-fiber diets and lower levels of inflammatory markers in the blood.

CAROTENOIDS: Found in carrots, garnet yams, squash, and cantaloupe, beta-carotene and other carotenoids appear to significantly reduce the risk of inflammatory arthritis.

VITAMIN K: Found in leafy greens like kale and chard, brussels sprouts, broccoli, cabbage, and seafood, vitamin K is a key nutrient that helps regulate the body's inflammatory processes. It's also a powerful antioxidant, so it reduces oxidative stress that can lead to inflammation.

MAGNESIUM: Found in green leafy vegetables, nuts, seeds, legumes, and whole grains, magnesium ranks among the highest on the list of minerals that appear to protect against inflammation.

Another important aspect of an anti-inflammatory diet is that it is a low glycemic way of eating, which means it doesn't cause blood sugar to spike and crash throughout the day. The typical American diet tends to be high in refined grains and sugar, and low in fiber. That combination leads to an excess of sugar (in the form of glucose) in the blood. When that occurs over a long period of time, our bodies can become insensitive to the insulin signal that helps us take the glucose up into our cells for fuel. As a result, there's excess glucose floating around in places it doesn't belong, sounding those alarm bells that trigger the inflammatory response.

What other lifestyle factors help reduce inflammation? Research suggests that moderate physical activity, meditation, and good sleep hygiene can reduce inflammation. Conversely, smoking and alcohol abuse increase inflammation.

⟫⟫ LESSONS FROM THE MEDITERRANEAN ⟪⟪

There's a lot to be learned from the traditional dietary habits of the people living in regions bordering the Mediterranean Sea. Most notably, meals consisting primarily of fresh fruits, vegetables, whole grains, legumes, nuts, seeds, and plenty of olive oil appear to have a tremendous impact on longevity and quality of life.

In the 1950s, an American researcher named Ancel Keys decided to embark on a cross-cultural study involving seven countries in four regions (United States, Northern Europe, Southern Europe, and Japan). He and his team of researchers looked at dietary and lifestyle habits and incidences of cardiovascular disease and mortality. The research supported his hypothesis that there is a correlation between phytonutrient-rich, low-cholesterol diets and a decreased risk of cardiovascular disease.

Continued research on various aspects of the Mediterranean diet provides us with more good reasons to adopt this style of eating in order to combat inflammation. In 2013, a long-term study on the Mediterranean diet was actually terminated after five years because the benefits were so clear that it was considered unethical to continue. The study compared a low-fat diet to a Mediterranean-style diet supplemented with either olive oil or nuts. Both of the Mediterranean-diet study groups had 30 percent reduced risk of heart attacks, strokes, and deaths from cardiovascular disease. And participants were even allowed to drink one glass of wine per day!

Dr. Walter Willett, chair of nutrition at Harvard School of Public Health, conducted a meta-analysis on the Mediterranean diet and concluded that "over 80 percent of coronary heart disease, 70 percent of stroke, and 90 percent of type 2 diabetes can be avoided by healthy food choices that are consistent with the traditional Mediterranean diet."

There is also research supporting the additional benefits of adopting an anti-inflammatory diet in relation to some other prevalent conditions, including:

METABOLIC SYNDROME: This is a precursor to diabetes and cardiovascular disease and a person is diagnosed when three out of five of the following symptoms are present: high blood glucose, high blood pressure, high triglycerides, low HDL (good cholesterol) levels, and excess abdominal fat. Some recent studies have demonstrated a 25 percent reduction in the prevalence of metabolic syndrome with adherence to a Mediterranean-style diet, which is similar to the effects of prescription medications (without any of the downsides).

ALZHEIMER'S DISEASE: In a study of over 1,400 seniors, those who adhered most closely to a Mediterranean-style diet had 48 percent lower risk of mental degeneration progressing to Alzheimer's.

CANCER: A study in southern Europe revealed that adherence to a traditional Mediterranean diet was associated with a 6 percent reduction in cancer (along with a 9 percent decrease in cardiovascular mortality and a 13 percent reduction in Parkinson's disease).

It's becoming clear that some of the most widely feared diseases share a common inflammatory component, which can be largely prevented through an anti-inflammatory diet. As we continue to learn more about the compounds in foods that either initiate or prevent an inflammatory response, we'll be able to make dietary decisions that help offset our genetic risk. In the meantime, we have lots of evidence that the foundational foods of a Mediterranean diet (olive oil, fish, nuts, seeds, fruits, vegetables, and whole grains) can stave off inflammatory diseases and keep us healthy and well.

Tools for Success

The key to a successful food plan is having the best foods available and knowing how to enjoy them in the right portions. The Anti-Inflammatory Plate will help you keep portions in check, and the pantry list provides the template you need to create a food environment that sets you up for success. These essential tools make it easier for you to eat in a way that nourishes and satisfies without feeling like you're on a diet.

⟫⟫⟫ THE ANTI-INFLAMMATORY PLATE ⟪⟪⟪

Forget about the food pyramids from your youth—the Anti-Inflammatory Plate visual that follows will give you guidance on how to construct the layout of your plate and meals in a way that supports your anti-inflammatory goals.

As you can see, vegetables occupy the most real estate on the plate. These comprise your most powerful delivery system for vitamins, minerals, antioxidants, and other phytonutrients that have been shown to decrease inflammation. There's also a place for colorful, antioxidant-rich fruits, and you can set aside concerns of too much sugar from these sources because most fruit is loaded with fiber, which helps slow down the blood sugar response. Just try to eat twice as many vegetables as fruits throughout the day.

Your portion of complex carbohydrates can be some of the starchier vegetables, like sweet potatoes and yams, carrots, and beets, or it can be from whole grains like brown rice or quinoa. Complex carbs are useful because they are what give us energy and help fuel our brain. It's also important when eating a more plant-based diet to include some whole grains in combination with beans to get your protein needs met. Speaking of protein, that section of the plate is smaller than what's customary for most Americans. The best bet for anti-inflammatory protein is fish, but grass-fed beef, bison, lamb, and free-range organic poultry are acceptable in small amounts. Vegetarian protein sources include legumes, nuts, seeds, and soy. Whole soy foods, such as edamame, tofu, tempeh, and miso, can be great additions to a plant-based diet. However, soy foods are not featured in this cookbook because all of the recipes provided are hypoallergenic, and soy is one of the top food allergens (but certainly not a problem for everyone!).

Finally, note that there's a place on the plate for fats and oils. It's time to let go of those fat phobias from the '80s and enjoy the delicious, satisfying healthy fats that complete an anti-inflammatory meal. These are primarily unsaturated fats and oils that often contain omega-3s and other phytosterols that are part of the anti-inflammatory pathways in the body. Including fat in your diet can also help you feel satiated and can help significantly decrease overeating.

The Anti-Inflammatory Plate

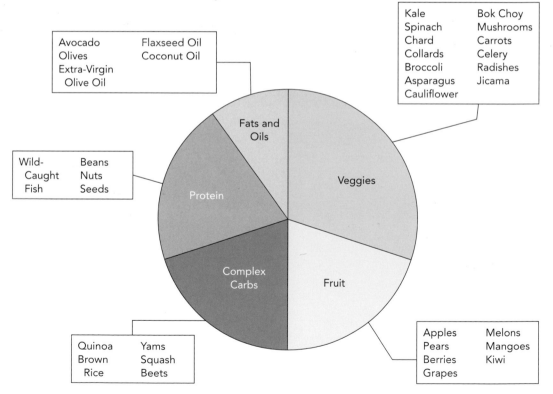

THE ANTI-INFLAMMATORY PANTRY

Keeping your pantry and fridge well stocked with foods that support your health and wellness goals is a big step in the right direction. By having the following items on hand, you'll be primed to quickly prepare anti-inflammatory recipes, and you'll avoid having to make a special trip to the store at the last minute. Many of the things listed can be stored for several weeks or more, so you shouldn't have any problem using them up well before the expiration dates.

MUST-HAVES	BENEFITS	USES	STORAGE
Fats and Oils			
Avocado oil	Great source of monounsaturated fat; more heat stable than olive oil	Frying, sautéing, roasting, grilling; dressings, marinades	Pantry
Coconut oil	Body uses this type of fat as energy; cholesterol-free	Sautéing; butter or shortening replacement	Pantry
Flaxseed oil	Plant-based source of omega-3s	Finishing only (do not heat); dressings, smoothies	Refrigerator
Grapeseed oil	Naturally stable oil that does not oxidize at higher temperatures	Frying, sautéing, roasting, grilling	Pantry
Extra-virgin olive oil	Great source of mono-unsaturated fat with unique antioxidant polyphenols that have anti-inflammatory properties	Light sautéing, finishing; dressings, marinades	Refrigerator or cool, dark pantry

MUST-HAVES	BENEFITS	USES	STORAGE
Nuts and Seeds			
Almonds	Contain healthy fats that decrease inflammation, help lower cholesterol; rich source of vitamin E	Snacking, topping (baked goods, salads, etc.); almond butter, almond milk	Airtight container in pantry
Flaxseeds	Excellent plant-based source of omega-3s, unique forms of fiber that improve digestion	Topping (baked goods, salads, etc.); smoothies; egg replacer	Sealed bag in refrigerator or freezer
Pumpkin seeds	Provide a very diverse blend of antioxidants; good source of magnesium, zinc, iron	Snacking, topping (baked goods, salads, etc.); pumpkin seed butter	Airtight container in pantry
Walnuts	Contains higher amounts of omega-3s than other nuts; rich in anti-inflammatory phytonutrients	Snacking, topping (baked goods, salads, etc.); dips, spreads	Airtight container in refrigerator or cool, dark pantry
Grains and Legumes			
Buckwheat (flour or groats)	Not actually a grain but a very nourishing fruit seed; gluten-free, so a good flour alternative for those avoiding wheat or gluten	Bean or grain dishes, soups, stews, salads; flour replacement	Flour: Sealed bag in freezer; Groats: Pantry
Legumes (adzuki, black, chickpea, lentils, navy, pinto)	Excellent source of fiber, particularly soluble fiber; valuable plant-based source of protein, essential nutrients; gluten-free	Bean or grain dishes, soups, stews, salads, dips	Pantry

MUST-HAVES	BENEFITS	USES	STORAGE
Quinoa (flour or whole)	The only grain considered a complete protein; contains small amounts of omega-3s; gluten-free	Bean or grain dishes, soups, stews, salads	Flour: Sealed bag in freezer; Whole: Pantry
Rice (flour or whole: black, brown, purple, red)	Excellent source of fiber, antioxidants that protect against type 2 diabetes and heart disease; gluten-free	Bean or grain dishes, soups, stews, salads	Flour: Sealed bag in freezer; Whole: Pantry
Herbs and Spices			
Cinnamon	Inhibits release of pro-inflammatory messengers in the body; helps regulate blood sugar	Fruit, oatmeal, smoothies, chili, stews	Pantry
Cumin	Stimulates digestive enzymes; contains cancer-preventing compounds	Beans, vegetables, chili, dips, marinades	Pantry
Ginger (dried or fresh)	Contains the anti-inflammatory compounds gingerols; immune-boosting properties	Smoothies, dressings, vegetables, desserts, teas	Dried: Pantry; Fresh: Refrigerator
Oregano (dried or fresh)	Excellent source of vitamin K, which helps regulate the body's inflammatory processes	Beans, vegetables, chili, dips, marinades	Dried: Pantry; Fresh: Refrigerator

continued

MUST-HAVES	BENEFITS	USES	STORAGE
Rosemary (dried or fresh)	Contains compounds that stimulate immune system, improve circulation, decrease inflammation	Beans, vegetables, chili, dips, marinades	Dried: Pantry; Fresh: Refrigerator
Turmeric (dried or fresh)	Contains curcumin and volatile oils that have powerful anti-inflammatory effects	Curries, soups, stews, rice, vegetables, lentils	Dried: Pantry; Fresh: Refrigerator

For most people, just stocking the pantry with the ingredients listed here and using the Anti-Inflammatory Plate as a model will be enough to start restoring balance to their bodies and transforming their health. Others need a more intensive overhaul to get them started on a new dietary path. The next chapter covers how to embark on a 21-day anti-inflammatory cleanse to do just that. While the majority of people report feeling better while on the cleanse, it's particularly useful for those who suffer from conditions like irritable bowel syndrome or digestive distress, osteo- or rheumatoid arthritis, congestion or sinusitis, and/or skin conditions such as eczema or psoriasis. The cleanse is definitely an optional course of action—read through the instructions and determine if it's the right fit for you. Otherwise feel free to skip straight ahead to the recipes and start cooking!

21-Day Nutritional Cleanse to Combat Inflammation

This is where the rubber meets the road. If you've been a victim of chronic inflammation for as long as you can remember, or you just want to get a handle on it before it becomes a problem, you can benefit from an anti-inflammatory cleanse. The key to a good cleanse is that it's supported with nutritionally robust foods that provide the body with key nutrients to heal. I'm not a proponent of fasting or juice cleanses as a method for reducing inflammation in the body. Results from those types of cleanses are fleeting at best.

In contrast, by following this 21-day plan, you'll discover how to nourish yourself with delicious whole foods that support optimal health. You'll be omitting foods that are most commonly associated with inflammation and those that are among the eight most allergenic foods. If you're having an immune response to something you're eating regularly, such as bread, cheese, or eggs, then you're accidentally keeping your body in an inflammatory state.

The 21-day program that I recommend is based on an elimination diet, which is the gold standard for diagnosing food allergies. In addition to the usual omissions, this plan also has you taking a break from vegetables in the nightshade category, including potatoes, tomatoes, peppers, and eggplant. While these foods are not pro-inflammatory for everyone, they do contain a compound called alkaloids, which some people have difficulty breaking down. I've had a number of patients with arthritis who claim that their symptoms get significantly worse during tomato season when they're harvesting their beautiful crops and eating tomatoes to their hearts' content.

The obvious reaction to an elimination diet of any kind is to focus on the foods that you can't eat. Those who have the best results and enjoy the lasting benefits of this nutritional cleanse are those who focus more on all of the fabulous, nourishing, anti-inflammatory foods that they *can* eat. Within Phase II,

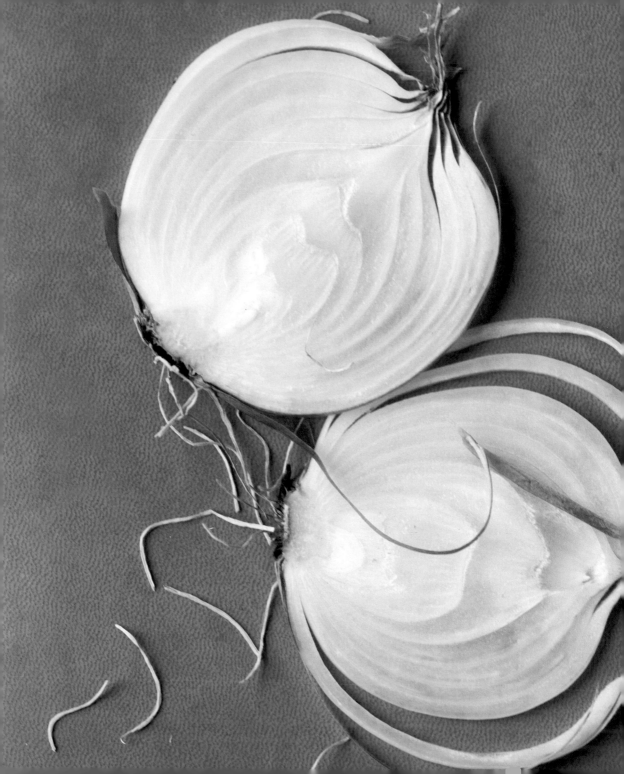

you'll find the list of foods to include and exclude during the cleanse, and I've highlighted some "best bet" foods that have specific properties known to squelch the inflammatory processes in the body. If you did nothing more than just add more of these best-bet foods to your daily diet, it's likely that you'll start to see a positive shift occurring.

⟶⟫ PHASE I: PREPARATION ⟪⟵

First, look at your calendar and find a one-month block without travel or too many social distractions—this is the ideal time to fit a cleanse into your schedule for optimal results. Then it's time to start preparing for the cleanse. I usually recommend giving yourself a full week to get your body and your pantry ready before you begin. For example, one of the most challenging parts of this cleanse for most people is giving up caffeine and sugar, so use this preparation week to help reduce dependence, which will in turn minimize unpleasant withdrawal symptoms.

What follows are some useful tips to help you feel stronger and more confident once you officially start your 21-day cleanse.

Reduce Caffeine

If you're consuming caffeine in any form, start weaning yourself now. If you drink coffee, go from caffeinated to half-decaf, to full decaf (preferably Swiss Water decaf), to green or black tea, and eventually to herbal tea. If you drink soda, switch to caffeine-free versions and then replace with water. For any other caffeine sources, gradually decrease the amount each day until you've removed it from your diet completely.

Start Drinking (Water, That Is!)

Start increasing your water intake so that you're drinking at least sixty to seventy ounces of water and/or herbal tea every day. This flushes out toxins and keeps you well hydrated, which can help abate some withdrawal symptoms.

Tame the Sugar Beast

Cut back on refined sugar and start reading the nutrition labels and ingredient lists on all packaged food products you buy to get in the habit of knowing exactly what's in your food. You'll be avoiding items that contain sugar, sucrose, evaporated cane juice, high fructose corn syrup, or any artificial sweeteners like sucralose or aspartame.

Stock Up on the Right Stuff

When you go shopping, go heavy on fruits, vegetables, beans, brown rice or quinoa, nuts, seeds, and fish. See the table on page 18 for specific ingredients to purchase (and avoid) for this cleanse.

Rev Up Your Metabolism

Get in the habit of eating a nutritious breakfast within one hour of rising and then have a small meal or healthy snack every three to four hours.

Get Your Act Together

Start making your meal plan and shopping list for the first week of the cleanse. It's a good idea to have your pantry and refrigerator fully stocked and to do some advance recipe prep, like washing and chopping vegetables, making a salad, and cooking up some quinoa or rice. Spending a few hours upfront will make the cleanse that much more enjoyable, keeping you stress-free and on track.

Finally, get ready to feel amazing!

⟫⟫⟫ PHASE II: NOURISH AND CLEANSE ⟪⟪⟪

For the next twenty-one days, you will be completely eliminating the top eight allergens (wheat/gluten, dairy, soy, eggs, corn, peanuts, shellfish, and oranges) from your diet. In addition, you'll leave behind caffeine, sugar, and alcohol. If you suffer from joint pain or any overt inflammatory condition (e.g. inflammatory bowel disease), you may also choose to omit the nightshade vegetables (potatoes, tomatoes, eggplant, and peppers) to see if those alkaloid-containing foods are exacerbating your symptoms.

So what *can* you eat? What's left is a very robust and anti-inflammatory Mediterranean-style diet. You'll be nourishing yourself with vegetables, fruits, nuts, seeds, legumes, gluten-free whole grains, finfish, and small amounts of organic meat and poultry. You definitely won't go hungry if you plan well. This book will be an invaluable resource because every recipe that's included is cleanse-friendly!

As you review the table that follows of foods to include and exclude, be sure to take note of the "best bets" column for each category. The best-bet foods contain phytonutrients and/or essential fatty acids that reverse the inflammatory processes in your body. These are the foods that you should intentionally try to eat more regularly, with a goal of including at least five of them from any category in your diet every day.

Foods to Include and Exclude on the Cleanse

	FOODS TO INCLUDE	BEST BETS	FOODS TO EXCLUDE
Vegetables	Fresh raw, steamed, sautéed, juiced, or roasted vegetables	Beets, broccoli, brussels sprouts, carrots, chard, kale, onions, spinach, garnet or jewel yams	Corn, creamed vegetables, nightshades (eggplant, peppers, potatoes, tomatoes)
Fruits	Fresh or frozen fruits, unsweetened fruit juices	Apples, avocados, berries, grapes, kiwis, melons, pears	Oranges, orange juice
Grains	Amaranth, buckwheat, millet, oats (certified gluten-free), quinoa, rice, tapioca, teff	Buckwheat, quinoa, rice (brown or red)	Barley, corn, gluten-containing products, kamut, rye, spelt, wheat
Animal Proteins: Fish and Meat	Fresh, frozen, or canned (water-packed) fish; small amounts of 100% grass-fed beef, wild game, lamb, free-range organic poultry	Wild-caught finfish: black cod, cod, halibut, salmon, sardines	Canned meats, cold cuts, eggs, frankfurters, pork, sausage, shellfish
Vegetable Proteins: Legumes	All beans (except soy), peas, lentils	Adzuki beans, black-eyed peas, hummus, lentils, mung beans	All soy products, including edamame, soy milk, tempeh, tofu
Fats	Almond, coconut, flaxseed, grapeseed, extra-virgin olive, pumpkin, safflower, sunflower, sesame, and walnut oils	Coconut oil, grapeseed oil, extra-virgin olive oil, olives	Butter, margarine, mayonnaise, processed and hydrogenated oils, shortening, spreads

	FOODS TO INCLUDE	BEST BETS	FOODS TO EXCLUDE
Nuts and Seeds	Almonds, cashews, walnuts; chia, pumpkin, sesame, and sunflower seeds; butters made from these nuts and seeds, tahini	Almonds, chia seeds, pumpkin seeds, walnuts	Peanuts, peanut butter
Spices, Condiments, and Confections	All spices, vinegar, mustard (grain-free, made from mustard seed and vinegar)	Cinnamon, garlic, ginger, oregano, rosemary, turmeric	Barbecue sauce, chocolate and chocolate sauce, chutney, cocoa, ketchup, relish, soy sauce, other condiments
Dairy and Milk Substitutes	Unsweetened almond, coconut, hemp, rice, and other nut or seed milks	Unsweetened almond, coconut, and hemp milks	Butter, cheese, cottage cheese, cow's milk, cream, frozen yogurt, ice cream, yogurt
Beverages	Filtered or distilled water, herbal tea, seltzer or mineral water	Herbal tea, water	Alcohol, coffee, all caffeinated and/or sweetened beverages
Sweeteners	Agave nectar, blackstrap molasses, coconut palm sugar, fruit sweetener, honey, pure maple syrup, stevia	Blackstrap molasses, coconut palm sugar, raw honey	Aspartame, corn syrup, evaporated cane juice, high-fructose corn syrup, refined sugar (white or brown), sucralose, other artificial sweeteners

Getting the Most From Your Cleanse

Here are some tips for a successful 21-day cleanse:

1. Eat breakfast within one hour of rising.

2. Eat a small meal or snack every three to four hours.

3. Put your eating emphasis on vegetables (focus on variety and lots of color!).
    - » Beets (raw, roasted, steamed)
    - » Cruciferous vegetables (broccoli, brussels sprouts, cabbage, cauliflower, kale)
    - » Garlic and onions
    - » Leafy greens (beet greens, chard, collard greens, dandelion greens, kale, spinach)

4. Eat anti-inflammatory sources of protein.
    - » Fish three to four times per week
    - » Vegetarian meals two to three times per week
    - » Other meat sources not more than one or two times per week (grass-fed beef, buffalo/bison, lamb, free-range organic poultry)

5. Eat plenty of good, healthy fats.
    - » Avocados
    - » Flaxseed oil
    - » Olives
    - » Raw nuts and seeds (lightly roasted is OK)

6. Eat at least five foods from the "best bets" column every day.

7. Stay well hydrated! Aim for sixty-four ounces of water and/or herbal tea every day (more if you're exercising).

8. Eat slowly and mindfully, focusing on the act of self-nourishment. Avoid watching TV, working on the computer, and other distractions while eating. Take three deep breaths before you start eating.

Menu Plans and Shopping Lists

The most challenging part of doing a cleanse (and eating healthy in general) is often the planning and prep. There are several ways you can approach this, and I always tell my clients to experiment until they find a routine that works within the context of their lives. The same goes for you. I've created a few different menus and accompanying shopping lists to accommodate a variety of eaters, including:

1. **MENU PLAN 1**: The Variety Lover—Perfect for the person who tires of leftovers quickly and enjoys experimenting with new recipes as part of the daily routine.

2. **MENU PLAN 2**: The Repeater—This menu is great for the person who says "I could eat the same thing every day, no problem!" It still adds some variety, but this menu requires far less cooking and fewer ingredients.

3. **MENU PLAN 3**: The Grain Avoider—If you feel like you tend to do better with no grains in your diet, this menu is for you. It's well-balanced yet completely devoid of all grains (even gluten-free ones).

You can choose the menu type that appeals most to you, or experiment with all three menus over the course of the 21-day cleanse. You can also use the menus to help guide you in your meal planning beyond the cleanse. You'll notice that balance and variety are key elements of menu planning. Snacks generally include a complex carbohydrate along with some type of protein and/or healthy fat. All meals have a healthy dose of fruits or vegetables along with some kind of protein.

What follows are a few dos and don'ts to help make your planning and food prep easier:

DO

» Choose foods you enjoy

» Make a plan before you shop

» Shop once or twice a week

» Carefully read ingredient lists on packaged foods

» Wash, chop, and prep your foods as you're putting away the groceries

» Use shortcuts (e.g. canned beans or pre-washed and chopped veggies)

» Make a couple recipes on your day off and freeze extra portions

» Pack snacks to take to work or to have in the car

» Let servers know what foods you're avoiding when dining out and ask for guidance

» Eat when you're hungry

» Eat slowly and mindfully, savoring every bite

DON'T

» Feel like you need to cook something new at every meal (unless you love to cook!)

» Allow yourself to get overly hungry

» Get caught up in calorie counting and restricting

» Assume that foods labeled as "gluten-free" or "all natural" are healthy by default

» Rely too heavily on rice or rice-based products for convenience—the objective is to eat lots of colorful, fresh foods

» Ignore your body's natural cues

Storage Tips

» Use a salad spinner to dry lettuce, wrap it in paper towels, and store in the crisper (no bag necessary).

» Store chopped carrots and celery in an airtight container full of water.

» Store fresh herbs in a small vase or glass that is half full of water (like a little bouquet!) and refrigerate.

» Slice wet vegetables, such as cucumbers, as needed instead of in advance.

» Use Debbie Meyer GreenBags to extend the life of your produce by a few days. The bags can be rinsed and reused multiple times.

» Invest in glass storage containers and get rid of the plastic.

» Reuse glass jars to store and freeze portions of soups and stews.

MENU PLAN #1: THE VARIETY LOVER

	MONDAY	TUESDAY	WEDNESDAY
BREAKFAST	Berry Green Power Smoothie	Mango Muesli with Brazil Nut Topping	Berry Green Power Smoothie
SNACK	Apple and 1 tablespoon almond or cashew butter	¼ cup pumpkin seeds	Pear and ¼ cup walnuts
LUNCH	Rainbow Quinoa with Roasted Asparagus and Adzuki Beans	Fish Taco Salad with Strawberry Avocado Salsa	Rainbow Quinoa with Roasted Asparagus and Adzuki Beans
SNACK	White Bean and Kalamata Olive Hummus and vegetables	Creamy Avocado Spinach Dip and vegetables	Anti-Inflammatory Trail Mix
DINNER	Poached White Fish with Mango Lime Chutney	Hearty Mushroom and Lentil Stew	Hearty Mushroom and Lentil Stew

THURSDAY	FRIDAY	SATURDAY	SUNDAY
Mango Muesli with Brazil Nut Topping	Berry Green Power Smoothie	Sweet or Savory Quinoa Crepes	Sweet Potato Hash with Lamb Sausage
Apple and 2 tablespoons White Bean and Kalamata Olive Hummus	Anti-Inflammatory Trail Mix	Nutty Coconut Energy Truffles	Berry Green Power Smoothie
Wilted Kale Salad with Shredded Beets and Carrots	Super Greens Salad with Pomegranate and Toasted Hazelnuts and leftover salmon	Super Greens Salad with Pomegranate and Toasted Hazelnuts	Leftover kale and chard with canned skipjack tuna
Artichoke and Basil Tapenade and celery	1 cup grapes and ¼ cup pistachios	Artichoke and Basil Tapenade and celery	Crispy Curried Chickpeas
Salmon en Papillote with Silky Celery Root Puree	Portobello Mushrooms with Samosa Filling and Wilted Kale Salad with Shredded Beets and Carrots	Pan-Fried Sardines with Sautéed Kale and Chard	Puttanesca-Style Beans and Greens

Fresh Produce

Apples, 2
Arugula, 5 cups
Asparagus, 1 pound
Avocados, 3
Banana, 1
Beets, 2
Carrots, 6
Celeriac (celery root),
    1 medium
Celery, 1 head
Chard, 3 bunches

Cremini mushrooms,
    ½ pound
Garlic, 2 heads
Garnet yams, 3
Ginger, 1 (1-inch) piece
Grapes, 1 bunch
Green onions, 2 bunches
Kale, 4 bunches
Lemons, 3
Limes, 2
Mango, 1
Pear, 1

Pomegranate, 1
Portobello mushrooms, 3
Red onion, 1
Shallots, 3 small
Shiitake mushrooms,
    1 pound
Spinach, 6 cups
Strawberries, 3
Sunchokes (Jerusalem
    artichokes), 4
Yellow onions, 3

Frozen Foods

Mango, 1 cup chopped

Mixed berries, 1 cup

Peas, ¾ cup

Fish, Meat, and Poultry

Anchovies, 4, or anchovy
    paste, 1 to
    2 teaspoons
Lamb sausages, 2
    (I recommend Uli's)

Light fish (cod, halibut, or
    red snapper),
    1½ pounds
Salmon, 1½ pounds
Sardines, 1 pound fresh

White fish (black cod,
    cod, or halibut),
    1½ pounds

Cereals, Grains, and Flours

Brown rice flour, ¾ cup

Oats, 1½ cups certified
    gluten-free

Quinoa flour, 2 cups
Rainbow quinoa, 1 cup

Nuts, Seeds, and Dried Fruits

Almond butter, ½ cup
Almonds, 1 cup raw
Blueberries, ½ cup
    freeze-dried
Brazil nuts, ½ cup
Cashews, ¾ cup raw
Cherries, ½ cup dried

Chia seeds, ¼ cup
Dates, ½ cup pitted
Hazelnuts, ¾ cup
Mangoes, ½ cup dried
    (unsweetened and
    unsulfured)
Pine nuts, ¼ cup

Pistachios, 1½ cups
    shelled
Pumpkin seeds (pepitas),
    1½ cups shelled
Tahini (sesame seed
    paste), 1 tablespoon
Walnuts, 2 cups

Herbs and Spices

Basil, 4 to 5 large leaves
   or 2 teaspoons dried
Bay leaf, 1
Black peppercorns
Cardamom, ½ teaspoon
   ground
Cayenne pepper,
   ⅛ teaspoon
Celery seed, 1 teaspoon
Cilantro, 1 bunch

Cinnamon, 2 tablespoons
   ground
Cumin, 1 tablespoon
   ground
Curry powder,
   2 teaspoons
Fenugreek, ½ teaspoon
   dried
Mint, 4 leaves
Nutmeg, ½ teaspoon
   ground

Oregano, 1 tablespoon
   fresh, or 2 teaspoons
   dried
Parsley, 1 bunch
Sage, 1 teaspoon dried
Sea salt
Thyme, 1 tablespoon
   fresh, or 2 teaspoons
   dried
Turmeric, 1 teaspoon
   ground

Oils and Vinegars

Balsamic vinegar,
   2 tablespoons
Champagne vinegar,
   1 tablespoon

Coconut oil, ¼ cup
Extra-virgin olive oil,
   1 (16-ounce) bottle

Grapeseed oil,
   1 (12-ounce) bottle
Sunflower oil (optional),
   1 tablespoon

Sweeteners

Agave nectar,
   3 teaspoons

Honey, 2 teaspoons

Maple syrup,
   2 tablespoons

Other

Adzuki beans,
   1 (15-ounce) can
Almond extract,
   ⅛ teaspoon
Almond milk, 1 cup
   unsweetened
Artichoke hearts mari-
   nated in olive oil,
   1 (14-ounce) jar
Baby lima beans, 1 cup
   dried
Baking powder,
   2 tablespoons
Baking soda, ½ teaspoon

Black beans,
   1 (15-ounce) can
Cannellini or other
   white beans,
   1 (15-ounce) can
Capers, 2 teaspoons
Chickpeas (garbanzo
   beans),
   1 (15-ounce) can
Coconut, ½ cup unsweet-
   ened and shredded
Coconut milk, 1 cup
   unsweetened

Cooking sherry,
   2 tablespoons
French lentils, ½ cup
   dried
Golden raisins, ¼ cup
Green olives, 1½ cups
Hemp milk (optional),
   ½ cup unsweetened
Kalamata olives, 3 cups
   pitted
Kombu (optional),
   1 (2-ounce) package
Mushroom broth, 1 quart
Vegetable broth, 6 cups

NOTE: Add desired Sweet or Savory Quinoa Crepe fillings to shopping list.

MENU PLAN #2: THE REPEATER

	MONDAY	TUESDAY	WEDNESDAY
BREAKFAST	Berry Green Power Smoothie	Mango Muesli with Brazil Nut Topping	Berry Green Power Smoothie
SNACK	Apple and 1 table-spoon almond or cashew butter	Pear and ¼ cup walnuts	Apple and 1 table-spoon almond or cashew butter
LUNCH	Mediterranean White Bean Soup	Mediterranean White Bean Soup	Mediterranean White Bean Soup
SNACK	Artichoke and Basil Tapenade and vegetables	¼ cup pumpkin seeds	Artichoke and Basil Tapenade and vegetables
DINNER	Hazelnut-Encrusted Halibut with Dipping Sauce	Toasted Pecan Quinoa Burgers	Toasted Pecan Quinoa Burgers

THURSDAY	FRIDAY	SATURDAY	SUNDAY
Mango Muesli with Brazil Nut Topping	Berry Green Power Smoothie	Power-Packed Granola with Currants and Chia Seeds and unsweetened almond milk	Power-Packed Granola with Currants and Chia Seeds and unsweetened almond milk
Pear and ¼ cup walnuts	Apple and 1 table-spoon almond or cashew butter	Mixed berries and ¼ cup pumpkin seeds	Mixed berries and ¼ cup pumpkin seeds
Spring Pea and Jicama Salad	Spring Pea and Jicama Salad	Wilted Kale Salad with Shredded Beets and Carrots and Caramelized Carrot Soup	Wilted Kale Salad with Shredded Beets and Carrots and Caramelized Carrot Soup
¼ cup pumpkin seeds	Artichoke and Basil Tapenade and vegetables	Crispy Curried Chickpeas	Crispy Curried Chickpeas
Pumpkin Coconut Curry with White Fish	Pumpkin Coconut Curry with White Fish	Spaghetti Squash Primavera with Basil Walnut Pesto	Spaghetti Squash Primavera with Basil Walnut Pesto

Fresh Produce

Apples, 2
Avocados, 2
Baby spinach or baby
    kale, 2 cups
Banana, 1
Beets, 2
Broccoli, 2 heads
Carrots, 14
Celery, 1 head
Chard, 1 bunch

Cremini mushrooms,
    1 pound
Fresh spinach, ½ pound
Garlic, 1 head
Ginger, 1 (1-inch piece)
Jicama, 1 small
Kaffir lime leaves, 5
    (or buy 2 limes for zest
    and juice if lime leaves
    are not available)

Kale, 2 bunches
Lemon, 1
Pears, 2
Radishes, 10
Red onion, 1 small
Scallions or green onions,
    1 bunch
Spaghetti squash, 1 small
Yellow onions, 2 small

Frozen Foods

Mangoes,
    1 (10-ounce) bag

Mixed berries,
    1 (10-ounce) bag

Petite peas,
    3 (10-ounce) bags

Fish, Meat, and Poultry

Halibut, 1½ pounds

White fish (black cod,
    cod, or halibut),
    1 pound

Cereals, Grains, and Flours

Brown rice, ¼ cup
Brown rice flour, ¼ cup

Oats, 5½ cups certified
    gluten-free

Quinoa, 1 cup

Nuts, Seeds, and Dried Fruits

Almond butter, ½ cup
Brazil nuts, ½ cup
Cashews, ¼ cup raw
Chia seeds, ½ cup
Currants, ½ cup dried

Hazelnuts, 1 cup
Pecans, ¾ cup
Pine nuts, ¼ cup
Pumpkin seeds (pepitas),
    1 cup shelled

Sesame seeds, ¼ raw
Sunflower seeds, ¾ cup
Walnuts, 1½ cups

Herbs and Spices

Basil, 4 to 5 leaves and
1 teaspoon dried
Black peppercorns
Cardamom, ½ teaspoon
ground
Cayenne pepper,
¼ teaspoon
Cinnamon, 1 teaspoon
ground

Cumin, 3 teaspoons
ground
Curry powder,
2 teaspoons
Dill, 1 teaspoon dried
Fenugreek, ½ teaspoon
dried
Italian herbs, ½ cup dried
Mint, 4 leaves

Nutmeg, ½ teaspoon
ground
Oregano, 1 teaspoon
dried
Sea salt
Turmeric, 1 teaspoon
ground

Oils and Vinegars

Apple cider vinegar,
1 tablespoon
Balsamic vinegar,
2 tablespoons

Coconut oil, ¾ cup
Extra-virgin olive oil,
1 (16-ounce) bottle

Grapeseed oil,
3 tablespoons

Sweeteners

Agave nectar, ¼ cup

Coconut palm sugar,
½ cup

Honey, 1½ teaspoons

Other

Artichoke hearts mari-
nated in olive oil,
1 (14-ounce) jar
Black beans, ½ cup
Cannellini beans,
1 (15-ounce) can
Chickpeas (garbanzo
beans),
1 (15-ounce) can

Coconut milk, 2 cups
Dijon or stone-ground
mustard, ½ teaspoon
Dill pickles,
1 (8-ounce) jar
Green olives, ½ cup
Hemp or almond milk,
½ cup unsweetened

Kalamata olives,
½ cup pitted
Pumpkin puree,
1 (15-ounce) can
Vegenaise, 1 cup soy-free
Vegetable broth, 4 quarts

MENU PLAN #3: THE GRAIN AVOIDER

	MONDAY	TUESDAY	WEDNESDAY
BREAKFAST	Berry Green Power Smoothie	Sweet Potato Hash with Lamb Sausage	Sweet Potato Hash with Lamb Sausage
SNACK	Apple and 1 tablespoon almond or cashew butter	Anti-Inflammatory Trail Mix	Pear and ¼ cup walnuts
LUNCH	Brussels Sprout Slaw and canned sardines	Black-Eyed Pea and Escarole Soup	Brussels Sprout Slaw and canned sardines
SNACK	Black Bean and Artichoke Hummus and vegetables	Creamy Avocado Spinach Dip and vegetables	Black Bean and Artichoke Hummus and vegetables
DINNER	Wilted Kale Salad with Shredded Beets and Carrots and grilled chicken breast	Salmon en Papillote with Silky Celery Root Puree and Wilted Kale Salad with Shredded Beets and Carrots	Zucchini Noodles with Pistachio Pesto and Black Lentils

THURSDAY	FRIDAY	SATURDAY	SUNDAY
Salmon lox and sautéed vegetables	Berry Green Power Smoothie	Fresh Berry Parfait with Coconut Cashew Cream	Salmon lox and sautéed vegeta-bles
¼ cup pumpkin seeds	Anti-Inflammatory Trail Mix	Nutty Coconut Energy Truffles	Berry Green Power Smoothie
Black-Eyed Pea and Escarole Soup	Brussels Sprout Slaw and leftover white fish	Hearty Mushroom and Lentil Stew	Hearty Mushroom and Lentil Stew
Apple and 1 table-spoon almond or cashew butter	Mixed berries and ¼ cup walnuts	Artichoke and Basil Tapenade and vegetables	Artichoke and Basil Tapenade and vegetables
Poached White Fish with Mango Lime Chutney and steamed broccoli	Zucchini Noodles with Pistachio Pesto and Black Lentils	Oven-Roasted Black Cod with Smashed Sweet Peas	Grilled chicken breast with leftover zucchini noodles

Fresh Produce

Apple, 1
Avocados, 2
Banana, 1
Beets, 2
Brussels sprouts,
⅓ pound
Carrots, 12
Celeriac (celery root),
1 medium
Celery, 1 head
Chard, 1 bunch
Cremini mushrooms,
½ pound

Escarole, 1 head
Garlic, 1 head
Garnet yams, 2
Ginger, 1 (1-inch) piece
Kale, 4 bunches
Leeks, 3 medium
Lemons, 2
Lime, 1
Mango, 1
Mixed berries, 2 cups
Pear, 1
Portobello mushroom, 1

Purple cabbage,
1 small head
Red onions, 2
Shallots, 3
Shiitake mushrooms,
1½ pounds
Spinach, 4 cups
Sunchokes (Jerusalem
artichokes), 4
White or yellow onions,
2 large
Zucchini, 3 medium

Frozen Foods

Butternut squash, 1 cup
cubed

Mixed berries, 1 cup
Sweet peas, 2 cups

Fish, Meat, and Poultry

Black cod, 2 pounds
Chicken breasts,
2 (4-ounce) boneless
and skinless (free-
range organic)

Lamb sausages, 2
(I recommend Uli's)
Salmon, 1½ pounds
White fish (black cod,
cod, or halibut),
1½ pounds

Nuts, Seeds, and Dried Fruits

Almond butter,
2 tablespoons
Almonds, 1 cup raw
Blueberries, ½ cup
freeze-dried
Cashews, 1¼ cups raw
Cherries, ½ cup dried
Chia seeds,
2 tablespoons

Dates, ½ cup pitted
Golden raisins, ½ cup
Mangoes, ½ cup dried
(unsweetened and
unsulfured)
Pine nuts, ¼ cup
Pistachios, 1¼ cups
shelled

Poppy seeds,
2 teaspoons
Pumpkin seeds (pepitas),
1½ cups shelled
Tahini (sesame seed
paste), 1 tablespoon
Walnuts, 2½ cups

Herbs and Spices

Basil leaves, 4 to 5
Bay leaf, 1
Black peppercorns
Celery seed, 1 teaspoon
Cilantro, 1 bunch
Cinnamon, 2 tablespoons
    ground

Cumin, 1 teaspoon
    ground
Italian herbs,
    1 tablespoon
Mint, 4 leaves
Oregano, 2 tablespoons
    fresh or 1 tablespoon
    dried

Parsley, 1 bunch
Sage, 1 teaspoon dried
Sea salt
Sweet paprika,
    1 teaspoon
Thyme, 2 tablespoons
    fresh or 1 tablespoon
    dried

Oils and Vinegars

Balsamic vinegar,
    2 tablespoons
Coconut oil,
    3 tablespoons
Cooking sherry,
    2 tablespoons

Extra-virgin olive oil,
    1 (16-ounce) bottle
Flaxseed oil,
    1 tablespoon
Rice wine vinegar,
    3 tablespoons

Sunflower oil,
    2 tablespoons
Toasted sesame oil,
    2 tablespoons

Sweeteners

Agave nectar,
    1 tablespoon

Honey, 3 teaspoons

Maple syrup (optional),
    2 tablespoons

Other

Almond extract,
    ⅛ teaspoon
Black beans,
    1 (15-ounce) can
Black lentils, ½ cup dried
Black-eyed peas, 1½ cups
    dried

Coconut milk, ½ cup
    unsweetened
Coconut, ½ cup unsweet-
    ened and shredded
French lentils, ½ cup
    dried
Green olives, ½ cup

Hemp or almond milk,
    ½ cup unsweetened
Kalamata olives, ½ cup
    pitted
Marinated artichoke
    hearts, 1 (14-ounce) jar
Mushroom broth, 1 quart
Vegetable broth, 3 quarts

Anti-Inflammatory Meal and Snack Ideas

BREAKFASTS

» Gluten-free oatmeal with nut butter, chia seeds, and coconut milk, sweetened with agave nectar or coconut palm sugar

» Sautéed vegetables over rice or quinoa with cashews and sunflower seeds

» *Butternut Squash and White Bean Soup (page 81)*

» Hummus, avocado, and vegetables wrapped in a brown rice tortilla

» Smoked salmon with sautéed mushrooms and kale

» *Power-Packed Granola with Currants and Chia Seeds (page 53)* with unsweetened almond or hemp milk and fresh fruit

SNACKS

» Hummus and assorted vegetables (carrots, celery, cucumbers, jicama, radishes, snap peas, zucchini)

» Celery spread with *Artichoke and Basil Tapenade (page 68)*

» Fruit with nuts or seeds or nut or seed butter (almond, cashew, sesame, sunflower, walnut)

» Shelled pumpkin seeds

» Beans and quinoa with mango salsa

» Sardines

LUNCHES

» Lentil soup served over quinoa or rice

» Bean, greens, and grain bowl: black, adzuki, cannellini, or pinto beans with kale, chard, or spinach over quinoa or rice; add avocado and/or Karam's garlic sauce

» Lettuce wraps of canned skipjack tuna mixed with Soy-Free Vegenaise

» Mediterranean platter of vegetables, hummus, olives, salmon, and marinated mushrooms

» Salad with mixed vegetables, grilled chicken, avocado, and vinaigrette dressing

DINNERS

» Poached salmon with *Wild Rice and Roasted Vegetables (page 97)*
» Brown rice tortillas with black or pinto beans, rice, shredded cabbage, shredded zucchini, and avocado
» Lamb, mushroom, and zucchini skewers and *Roasted Cauliflower Soup with Gremolata (page 78)*
» Vegetarian stir-fry with toasted sesame oil and fresh ginger
» Bison burgers with oven-roasted sweet potato fries and mixed green salad
» Roasted free-range chicken with brussels sprouts and sweet potatoes

A note on portion control:

As a nutritionist who encourages mindful, intuitive eating, I am not a huge proponent of weighing and measuring every morsel of food that goes into your mouth. Generally speaking, when my clients start eating a variety of whole foods and limit or omit processed foods, portion control issues start to disappear. If you're obeying your hunger and satiety cues and eating slowly and mindfully that might be enough for you to self regulate. With that being said, it's quite possible to have too much of a good thing. There are some perfectly healthy whole foods that are calorically dense and portion awareness may be useful. Following are some serving size guidelines for some of those foods:

» Nuts and seeds = ¼ cup
» Nut and seed butters = 1 tablespoon
» Avocado = ¼ of a large avocado
» Grains (rice, quinoa, etc.) = ½ cup cooked
» Oatmeal = ¾ cup cooked
» Beans = ½ cup
» Hummus = ¼ cup

PHASE III: REINTRODUCTION

After enjoying three full weeks of clean eating and blissful nourishment, you might be feeling so good that you don't want to change a thing. While it's a good sign that you're still feeling enthusiastic about healthy eating as you approach the end of the cleanse, it's also important to remember that some of the foods you omitted during Phase II are perfectly great options. Let's take soy for example: If it's well tolerated and you plan to follow a more plant-based diet, whole soy foods like tofu, tempeh, and edamame can be a great way to get protein, calcium, and a host of other phytonutrients.

There are a couple options for reintroducing foods during this third phase. You can choose a less structured, slow reintroduction of the foods that you've been avoiding, or you may elect to do more formal food challenges. The latter is designed for those who are suspicious they might have specific food allergies or intolerances. When my clients have severe digestive disorders or skin issues that completely resolve during a cleanse, I typically suggest that they do formal food reintroductions to pinpoint which food or foods might be causing the symptoms.

Regardless of the option you choose, remember that you want to continue to build on your success and keep some of the healthy habits you've adopted. You also want to avoid shocking your squeaky clean system by bombarding your body with everything you've been avoiding in one fell swoop. It's generally not a good idea to celebrate the end of a cleanse with a large meat pizza, a pitcher of beer, and an ice cream sundae.

Option 1: Gentle Food Reintroduction (Less Structured)

1. Gradually ease foods back into your diet while holding strong to healthy eating habits (such as eating more vegetables and fresh, whole foods).

2. Try to limit food reintroductions to one new food group per day, and keep portion sizes reasonable (e.g., challenge dairy by having some plain yogurt with fruit and see how that goes).

3. Keep a journal to log any changes in how you're feeling as you introduce foods back into your diet. If there are any foods that aggravate your system in some way, this will help you connect the dots.

Option 2: Formal Food Reintroductions (More Structured)

1. Decide which food group to reintroduce first:
   » Wheat/gluten
   » Dairy
   » Eggs
   » Soy
   » Corn
   » Peanuts
   » Citrus
   » Nightshades (eggplant, peppers, potatoes, tomatoes)
   » Optional: Caffeine, sugar, and alcohol (challenge these substances if you want to see how sensitive you are, but generally it's just good practice to enjoy them in moderation, if at all)

2. Eat two or three average-size portions of a pure form of foods from that group through the course of one day. A pure form would mean that the food does not have additives or other ingredients that you have been omitting from your diet (e.g., sugar). Some examples of pure foods from some of the groups:
   » Wheat/gluten—Whole wheat tortilla (read ingredients), whole wheat pasta
   » Dairy—Milk, cheese without added color or flavor, plain yogurt

» Soy—Edamame, tempeh, plain soy milk (Eden or other brand that contains only filtered soybeans and water)

3. After one day of eating from that food group, remove it from your diet again. *You will keep this food group out of your diet through the end of the reintroduction phase, regardless of your reaction.* Observe how you feel for two days, which gives you time to notice both immediate and delayed reactions. Use a journal or notebook to record the foods you're challenging and record any potential reactions—write down anything that is at all different from when you were in the full elimination phase of the diet. Examples of potentials reactions include:
   » Skin irritations or break outs
   » Gas, bloating, or abdominal pain
   » Diarrhea or constipation
   » Headache
   » Fatigue, depression, or anxiety
   » Muscle or joint pain

4. *If you don't have any symptoms after two days,* reintroduce the next food group. Remember that you are challenging each group individually, so be sure to remove the food group from your diet after challenging it *even if you have no reaction* until you've completed all food reintroductions. *If you do have symptoms after challenging a food,* stop eating that food and allow the symptoms to clear completely before starting the next challenge.

5. Repeat steps two through four for each food group.

→→→ PHASE IV: TRANSITION TO LONG-TERM ANTI-INFLAMMATORY EATING ←←←

Once you've completed your 21-day nutritional cleanse and made your way through the food reintroductions, you'll want to identify habits that are worth continuing, hopefully for a lifetime. I always tell my clients that this shouldn't be viewed as a short-term "Hollywood cleanse." The goal is set your body straight and stay on the path to wellness. If you find you're in a rush to return to some favorite inflammatory foods (processed, sugary treats or excess meat), just remind yourself of the many ways in which you benefited from a clean diet: more energy, a change in body composition, less achiness and joint pain, a glowing complexion, and the like.

Here are some tips to help you stay on track post-cleanse:

» Make a weekly or monthly food plan—healthy eating doesn't just happen!

» Follow Michael Pollan's advice: "Eat food. Mostly plants. Not too much."

» Eat twice as many vegetables as fruits.

» Tame that sugar beast (mostly by avoiding refined sugar).

» Choose whole grains over avoid highly processed flour products.

» Reduce your consumption of processed foods by packing your own lunches and snacks.

» Find joy in *movement!* Be creative with exercise.

» Take several moments each day to breathe, relax, and regroup.

» Create a bedtime ritual and aim for seven to nine hours of sleep every night.

» Be kind, patient, and loving toward yourself. Change is not easy!

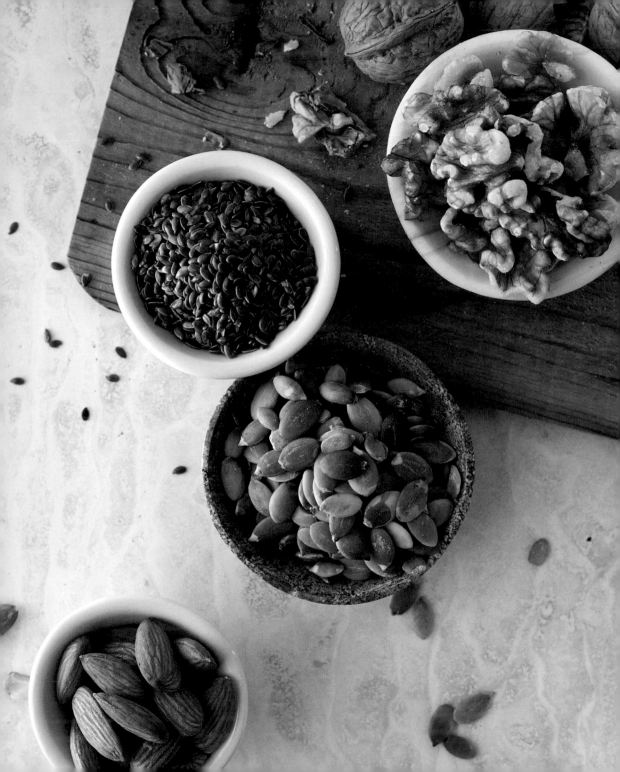

Breakfasts

What your mother always told you about breakfast is true. It really is the most important meal of the day. It brings you out of a fasting state, helps stabilize your blood sugar, and gives you the energy you need to face the day. Sadly, breakfast is still the most neglected meal. Busy schedules, sleep deprivation, lack of hunger cues, and a deficit of creative breakfast ideas are just a few of the reasons people give for skipping breakfast.

Well, friends, I'm happy to tell you that a little bit of planning and a few good recipes can help transform the chronic breakfast avoider into someone who springs out of bed in anticipation of that morning meal. If you're just getting used to the idea of having breakfast, start small. You might even find some of the snack ideas in the next chapter more appealing. If you just want to improve the quality of your breakfast, be sure to include some protein, complex carbs, and healthy fats in each morning meal. If you can start the day with a savory breakfast that includes vegetables, you'll be off to a winning start!

Breakfast Burrito with Chickpeas and Avocado

If you find yourself in a time crunch, and cooking in the morning is out of the question, this is the ideal savory breakfast. The chickpea-avocado combo makes a delicious burrito filling, and you can amp up the nutritional profile by adding your favorite greens. The sunflower seeds provide some crunch and a little extra protein. If you have leftover filling, you can have it for breakfast the next morning or use it as a dip. The avocado will discolor, but the taste will be just fine.

Makes 2 servings

1 (15-ounce) can of chickpeas, rinsed and drained
1 avocado
1 tablespoon freshly squeezed lemon juice
1 teaspoon sea salt
½ teaspoon ground cumin
½ teaspoon ground turmeric
2 tablespoons sunflower seeds
2 brown rice or teff tortillas
1 cup arugula, watercress, or microgreens

Put the chickpeas in a medium mixing bowl. Scoop the avocado into the bowl. Add the lemon juice, salt, cumin, and turmeric. Mash the mixture with a fork until the avocado is well incorporated. Allow some of the chickpeas to remain whole. Stir in the sunflower seeds.

Just before serving, sprinkle the tortillas with water and heat in the microwave for 20 seconds. Scoop half of the chickpea mixture into the center of each tortilla. Top with the arugula and roll up the tortillas like burritos.

The unique combination of healthy fats and phytosterols in avocados are what make them one of the top anti-inflammatory fruits. They are particularly useful in cooling down inflammation related to arthritis.

Smoked Salmon and Avocado Tartine

There's nothing like a savory open-faced sandwich after a long red-eye flight from coast to coast. I was nearly falling asleep in my latte at a French café in New York City, when I spotted a breakfast tartine amidst all the crepes and croissants on the menu. I felt myself come back to life as I polished off the tartine, and it inspired me to think up an endless combination of sandwich ingredients that would be suitable for breakfast.

If this breakfast can resurrect a person with severe jet lag, imagine what it will do for the average early riser. I refer to this tartine as the breakfast of champions because it's the perfect combination of carbohydrate, protein, and healthy fat.

Makes 4 servings

1 avocado
1 tablespoon freshly squeezed
   lime juice
1 teaspoon ground cumin
½ teaspoon sea salt

4 slices gluten-free bread, cut
   into quarters
8 ounces smoked salmon or lox
1 cup alfalfa sprouts or microgreens
4 radishes, thinly sliced

Scoop the avocado into a medium bowl. Add the lime juice, cumin, and salt and mash with a fork until the ingredients are well combined but the mixture is still chunky.

Arrange 4 bread pieces on each serving plate. Spread a layer of avocado mixture on each piece. Top with ½ ounce salmon. Stack some sprouts on the salmon and garnish with radish slices.

Salmon is an excellent source of anti-inflammatory omega-3s. Avocados are loaded with specific phyto-nutrients that block the inflammatory response and can decrease arthritic symptoms.

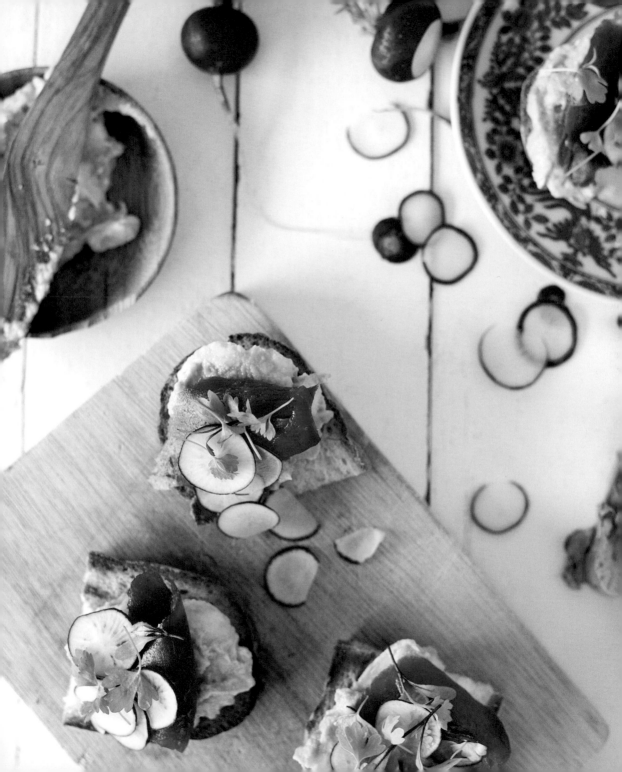

Breakfast Rice with Crumbled Nori

A recipe that naturopath Dr. Katherine Oldfield gives her patients inspired this quick and easy breakfast. It also happens to be a great way to clean out the refrigerator when you have leftover rice and soon-to-expire veggies in the produce bin. Anything goes in this breakfast sauté, so don't be afraid to add more vegetables and a different combination of nuts and seeds. It's also delightful when topped with a poached egg or some leftover salmon.

Makes 4 servings

1 tablespoon raw sesame seeds
2 teaspoons coconut oil
2 cloves garlic, crushed
1 shallot, chopped
6 cremini or button mushrooms, chopped
1 teaspoon sea salt
1 cup roughly chopped kale
1½ cups cooked brown rice (leftover rice works great!)
2 teaspoons toasted sesame oil
2 teaspoons mirin
¼ cup chopped raw cashews
2 tablespoons crumbled nori

Place a large sauté pan over medium heat. Add the sesame seeds to quickly toast until lightly browned, about 1 minute. Add the oil, garlic, and shallot and cook, stirring occasionally, until soft and fragrant, 3 to 4 minutes. Add the mushrooms and salt and sauté until tender, about 3 minutes. Fold in the kale and continue stirring until it starts to wilt, 3 to 4 minutes.

Stir in the rice, sesame oil, and mirin and cook until the rice is heated through, about 2 minutes. Top with the cashews and nori.

Sweet Potato Hash with Lamb Sausage

Brunch is one of my absolute favorite meals to host, and this dish is a hit every time I serve it. The key is thinly slicing the onions and leaving them in half rings so that they caramelize perfectly and create an amazing texture. You can use any type of sausage, but I much prefer using lamb. Not only does it have an impressive nutritional profile, but it also lends rich, complex flavors and blends perfectly with the sweetness of the garnet yams.

Makes 6 servings

2 lamb sausages (I recommend Uli's)
1 large white or yellow onion, thinly sliced into half rings
1 to 2 teaspoons sunflower oil (optional)
1 cup chopped cremini mushrooms
2 cloves garlic, minced

2 unpeeled garnet yams, cut into ¼-inch cubes
1 cup finely chopped kale
1 tablespoon fresh thyme
1 tablespoon fresh oregano
1 teaspoon ground sage
1 teaspoon sea salt
1 teaspoon freshly ground black pepper

Preheat the oven to 375 degrees F.

Squeeze the lamb out of its casing into a large cast-iron skillet over medium heat. As it cooks, break the lamb into small pieces with a spatula and sauté until it begins to brown, about 4 minutes. If using a leaner sausage, such as chicken, you may need to add some grapeseed or sunflower oil to the pan. With a slotted spoon, transfer the sausage to a bowl.

Add the onion to the skillet and sauté until it begins to caramelize, 4 to 5 minutes. Drizzle in sunflower oil as needed. Add the mushrooms and garlic and cook until softened, about three minutes. Stir in the yams, kale, thyme, oregano, sage, salt, and pepper and return the sausage to the skillet.

Transfer the skillet to the oven and roast for 20 to 25 minutes, or until the yams can be easily pierced with a fork.

Sweet or Savory Quinoa Crepes

One of my preferred pastimes is to chef it up with my good friend and mentor Barb Schiltz. Barb happens to be a masterful nutritionist and a longtime crepe lover, so we worked on this creation together and came up with a delicate but hearty crepe recipe. I prefer savory crepes and Barb prefers sweet, so I offer variations for both. Unless you have a special crepe pan, I find it easier to make smaller crepes (about three inches in diameter) and then stack the crepes with layers of filling in between.

Makes 6 servings

2 cups quinoa flour
2 tablespoons baking powder
½ teaspoon baking soda
¼ teaspoon sea salt
½ cup raw cashews
2 tablespoons chia seeds
1¾ cups water
1 cup unsweetened almond milk
2 tablespoons coconut oil
1 teaspoon freshly squeezed
    lemon juice
1 teaspoon maple syrup
Nonstick olive oil cooking spray

SWEET FILLING OPTIONS
2½ cups fresh or frozen berries
    (thawed if frozen)
2½ cups stewed apples or pears with
    cinnamon
2 cups cashew cream (1½ cups raw
    cashews blended with ½ cup water)
2½ cups mangoes blended with
    coconut milk

SAVORY FILLING OPTIONS
2½ cups sautéed onions, mushrooms,
    and spinach
2 cups hummus and 1 sliced avocado
2 ounces lox and 1 tablespoon capers

Whisk the flour, baking powder, baking soda, and salt in a medium mixing bowl and set aside. In a food processor or blender, grind the cashews and chia seeds until finely ground. Add the water, almond milk, oil, lemon juice, and maple syrup and blend for 2 to 3 minutes. Add the mixture to the dry ingredients, stirring until well blended. The batter should be the consistency of olive oil. Add more water to thin if necessary.

Spray a medium nonstick pan, cast-iron skillet, or crepe pan with oil. Put 2 to 3 table-spoons of the crepe batter in the pan and swirl around until there is a thin layer across the bottom. Cook each crepe for 1 minute per side. Fill with the desired filling.

Mango Muesli with Brazil Nut Topping

There's nothing better than waking up to find breakfast waiting for you in the fridge (except for maybe breakfast being served to you in bed!). I much prefer the texture of soaked oats to that of cooked porridge. The combination of mangoes with coconut milk gives this hearty cereal an exotic, tropical flair. And although Brazil nuts are commonly the ones that get left behind in the mixed nut dish, they're loaded with nutrients and good, healthy fats, making them a great topping for your muesli! Traditional muesli is served with yogurt; if you're avoiding dairy, you could try coconut, almond, or soy yogurt. It's also delicious with just the coconut milk.

Makes 4 servings

1½ cups certified gluten-free oats
2 cups water
1 cup coconut milk, plus more
for serving
1 cup chopped mango (thawed
frozen mango is OK)

1 teaspoon ground cinnamon
½ teaspoon ground nutmeg
½ teaspoon ground cardamom
½ cup roughly chopped Brazil nuts

In a large bowl with a lid, combine the oats, water, coconut milk, mango, cinnamon, nutmeg, and cardamom and stir well. Cover and place in the refrigerator for at least 4 hours or overnight. Serve with additional coconut milk or yogurt and sprinkle with Brazil nuts.

> Brazil nuts are a rich source of anti-inflammatory unsaturated fats. They're also an excellent source of selenium, a powerful antioxidant that helps optimize thyroid function.

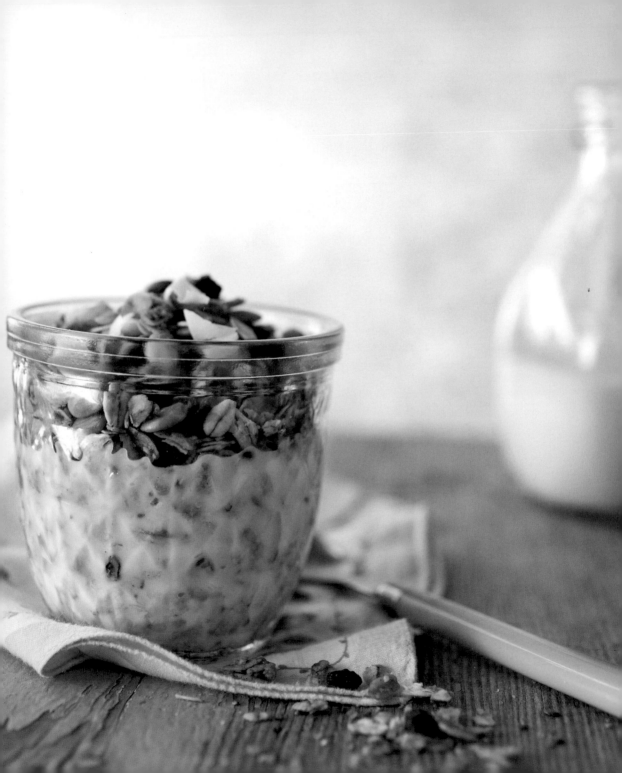

Power-Packed Granola with Currants and Chia Seeds

Part of my regular Sunday ritual is to make this granola and pop it into the oven first thing in the morning. I sit down with a cup of tea, watch the news, and take in the mouthwatering aroma that's reminiscent of oatmeal cookies. The timer dings, I salivate like I'm in a Pavlovian experiment, and then I enjoy a nice, warm bowl of granola. Store-bought granola is often loaded with sugar, but this recipe uses low-glycemic sweeteners and is high in protein. If you're a cereal lover, you can feel good about starting your day with this power-packed granola.

Makes 6 servings

4 cups certified gluten-free rolled oats

3 tablespoons chia seeds (I recommend Qia—a blend of chia, buckwheat, and hemp seeds)

¼ cup coconut palm sugar

¼ cup agave nectar

¼ cup coconut oil

2 tablespoons almond butter

½ cup dried currants

OPTIONAL ADDITIONS

½ cup chopped pecans

½ cup shelled pumpkin seeds (pepitas)

¾ cup unsweetened coconut flakes

½ cup raisins

½ cup dried cherries

Preheat the oven to 300 degrees F and line a baking pan with parchment paper.

In a large bowl, combine the oats, chia seeds, sugar, agave, oil, and almond butter and mix thoroughly. Spread the mixture evenly on the pan. Bake for 40 minutes, stirring after 20 minutes.

Allow the granola to cool completely before stirring in the currants and transferring to an airtight container.

Fresh Berry Parfait with Coconut Cashew Cream

I make coconut cashew cream as a fruit dip whenever I host brunch at my house, and people go crazy over it. They're always astonished when I tell them it's made from just cashews and coconut milk. Raw cashews have a wonderfully subtle sweetness and just the right amount of fat. They can easily be transformed into a perfect stand-in for whipped cream—particularly when you add coconut milk! Layering this creamy cashew goodness with fresh berries or mangoes creates a beautiful, satisfying breakfast that is loaded with antioxidants.

Makes 2 servings

1 cup raw cashews
½ cup unsweetened coconut milk
2 teaspoons honey
1 teaspoon ground cinnamon

2 cups berries (blackberries, blueberries, raspberries, strawberries—any combination works!)

Place the cashews, coconut milk, honey, and cinnamon in a food processor. Blend until smooth—the mixture should resemble creamy peanut butter. If it's too thick, slowly drizzle in some water and blend until it reaches the desired consistency.

Scoop two large spoonfuls of the cashew cream into the bottom of a small parfait glass. Add ½ cup of the berries and top with another layer of cashew cream. Finish with another ½ cup berries. Repeat in a second parfait glass.

Tip: The parfaits can be made ahead of time and stored in the refrigerator for 3 or 4 days for a ready-to-grab breakfast or a healthy-yet-decadent dessert.

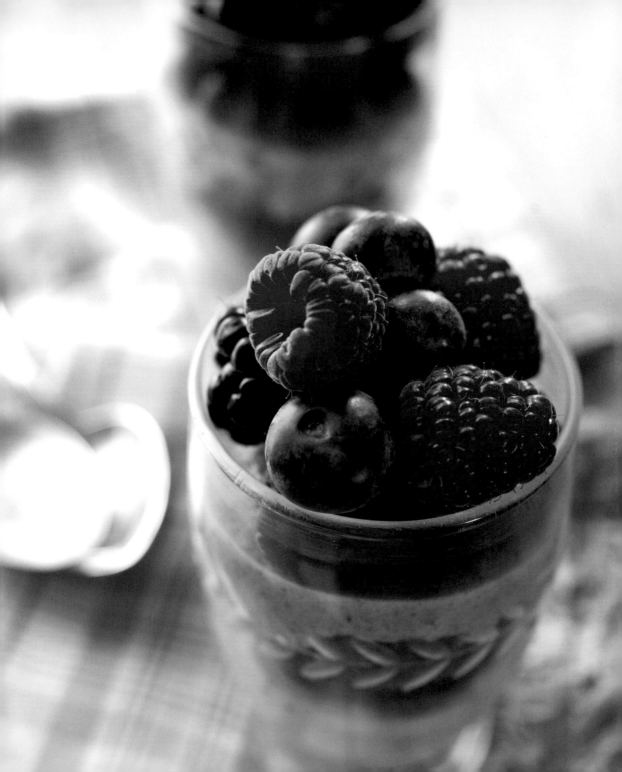

Berry Green Power Smoothie

Smoothies can be a great way to get several servings of fruits and vegetables without lifting a fork. There's no shortage of smoothie recipes, and it can be fun to experiment with different combinations. Just be sure that you're including a variety of colorful foods, some form of protein, and a little healthy fat to keep you satiated. This smoothie has some anti-inflammatory fresh herbs that help tone down the greens and brighten up the rest of the ingredients. I think it's pure bliss in a glass!

Makes 1 serving

2 cups spinach and/or baby kale
1 cup frozen mixed berries
½ banana
¼ cup raw cashews
4 mint leaves
2 tablespoons chia seeds

¾ cup water
½ cup unsweetened hemp or
   almond milk
1 teaspoon honey
¼ teaspoon minced fresh ginger

Toss all the ingredients in a blender, blend thoroughly, and enjoy!

> Ginger contains anti-inflammatory compounds called gingerols and also has immune-boosting properties, so it's a great safeguard during cold and flu season.

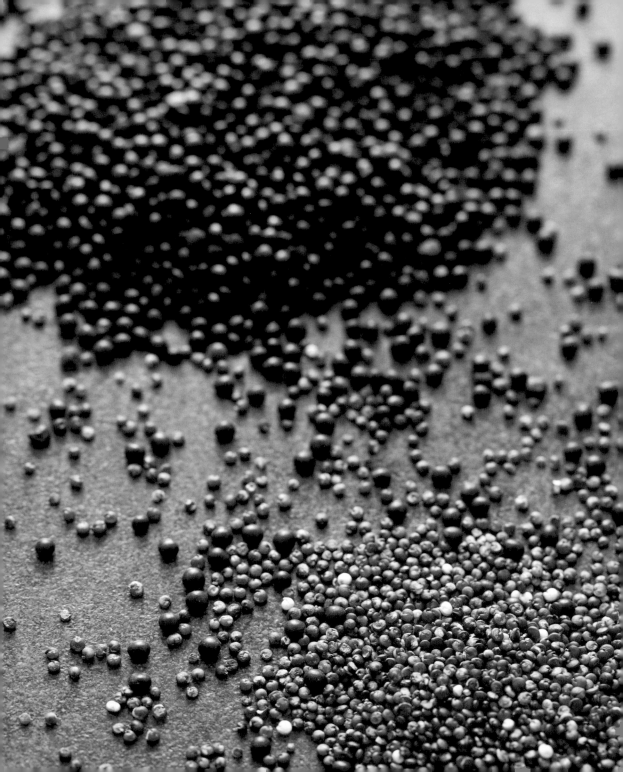

Healthy Snacks

Forget what you've heard about not snacking between meals. A well-planned snack in the afternoon might be just what the doctor ordered. Not only does it help keep your energy level up, but it also gives you another opportunity to work some nourishing anti-inflammatory foods into your daily diet. And if you avoid a blood sugar crash in the afternoon, you'll be much less likely to reach for the pro-inflammatory foods that are loaded with sugar.

A general rule of thumb is to avoid going more than four hours without eating. You should also be very intentional about fueling your body before workouts and replenishing it afterward. The snacks featured in this chapter are nourishing, well balanced, and can help reduce sugar cravings. I recommend preparing a few snack recipes on the weekend so you've got ready-made options to get you through the week. I also love the idea of setting out a dip with some veggies so the whole family can munch on something healthy while dinner is cooking.

Black Bean and Artichoke Hummus

I have to credit my sister for being the one who introduced me to the idea of adding artichoke hearts to a more traditional black bean dip, and it sure makes things more interesting! Use artichoke hearts marinated in olive oil to give this hummus a smoother finish and a richer flavor. I've also been known to stir in some fire-roasted peppers or sun-dried tomatoes for a slightly different twist on this dip.

Makes 6 servings

1 (15-ounce) can black beans, rinsed and drained

1 (6-ounce) jar artichoke hearts marinated in olive oil

2 cloves garlic, minced

1 tablespoon tahini

3 tablespoons extra-virgin olive oil

1 teaspoon sea salt

Place the beans, artichokes with oil, garlic, and tahini in a food processor. With the machine running, slowly drizzle in the oil and blend to the desired consistency. Season with the salt.

Serve with assorted vegetables, such as carrots, snap peas, cucumbers, zucchini, jicama, or daikon radishes.

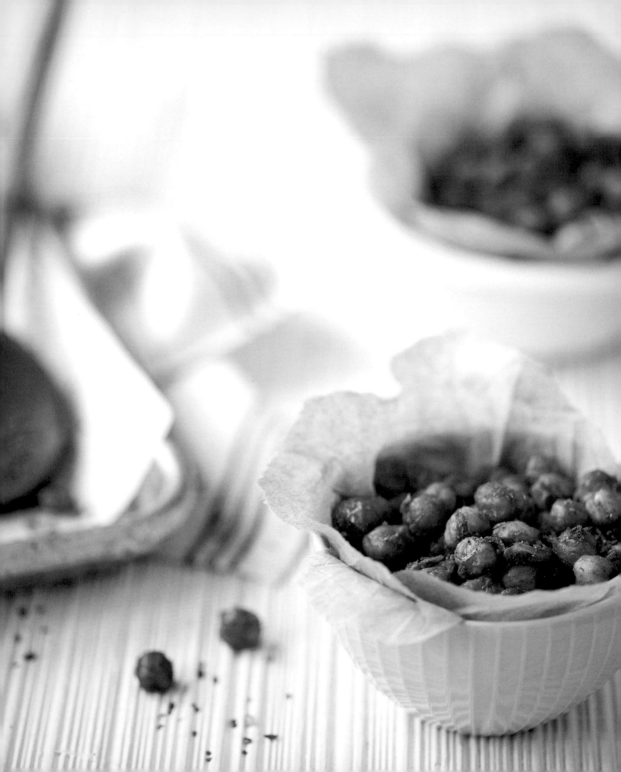

Crispy Curried Chickpeas

This is such an easy and nutritious snack to make! Chickpeas (also called garbanzo beans) are a good source of protein, and they're rich in iron and potassium. But what you'll notice most is that these crispy chickpeas really hit the spot when you're in the mood for a crunchy, salty snack! You can get creative with the seasonings and experiment with different herbs and spices.

Makes 4 servings

1 (15-ounce) can chickpeas, rinsed
    and drained
1 tablespoon grapeseed oil
2 teaspoons ground cumin
1 teaspoon ground turmeric

1 teaspoon sea salt
½ teaspoon freshly ground
    black pepper
½ teaspoon fenugreek

Preheat the oven to 400 degrees F.

Pat the chickpeas dry with a paper towel, then place in a medium bowl. In a small bowl, combine the oil, cumin, turmeric, salt, pepper, and fenugreek and whisk with a fork. Pour the oil mixture over the chickpeas and stir until they're well coated.

Spread the chickpeas on a baking pan and bake for 40 minutes, or until they're golden brown and rattle around the pan. Serve immediately, or cool thoroughly before storing in an airtight container.

Tip: These chickpeas are actually best when eaten shortly after cooking. They tend to lose some of their crispiness after storing unless the container is completely airtight.

White Bean and Kalamata Olive Hummus

Hummus is a great snack, but it's easy to get burned out on the traditional chickpea variety. Using white beans is a simple way to change it up enough that hummus will once again become exciting and new. White beans also have a more neutral flavor than chickpeas, so even those who generally dislike hummus often enjoy this version. White bean hummus can also be a more nutritious substitute for mayo and works great as a spread on vegetarian sandwiches.

Makes 6 servings

1 (15-ounce can) cannellini or other white beans, rinsed and drained
2 cloves garlic
1 tablespoon tahini

3 tablespoons extra-virgin olive oil
¼ cup pitted kalamata olives
1 teaspoon sea salt

Place the beans, garlic, and tahini in a food processor. With the machine running, slowly drizzle in the oil and blend to the desired consistency. Add the olives and pulse until they are just chopped and incorporated. Season with the salt.

Serve with assorted vegetables, such as carrots, snap peas, cucumbers, zucchini, jicama, or daikon radishes. The hummus can be stored in an airtight container in the refrigerator for up to 5 days.

Specific compounds in olives, called polyphenols, have been shown to block inflammatory pathways and reduce specific markers that are used to measure inflammation in the body.

Shiitake Mushroom and Walnut Pâté

If you like the idea of pâté, but are not a fan of liver, this recipe is for you. Toasting the walnuts illuminates their sweetness and tones down the bitter quality of their skins. You can use any type of mushrooms or a combination of different types (such as chanterelle, oyster, or morel). Including butter beans helps create a silkier texture and also adds some fiber and nutrients.

Makes 6 servings

1 cup raw walnuts
1 tablespoon coconut oil
6 shiitake mushrooms, sliced
¾ teaspoon sea salt, divided

½ cup cooked butter beans or other white beans (canned is OK)
1 teaspoon maple syrup

Preheat the oven to 350 degrees F.

Spread the walnuts on a baking pan and bake for about 12 minutes, or until they start to brown and get fragrant. Set aside.

In a small sauté pan, heat the oil. Add the mushrooms, season with ¼ teaspoon of the salt, and cook, stirring occasionally, until the mushrooms are soft and juicy, about 5 minutes.

Combine the walnuts, mushrooms, beans, maple syrup, and remaining ½ teaspoon salt in a food processor and blend until smooth. The mixture will be somewhat thick and will resemble liver pâté.

Serve with assorted vegetables or rice crackers.

> Walnuts are one of the few plant-based foods that contain an appreciable amount of omega-3s. They also contain some rare anti-inflammatory nutrients that are found in virtually no other commonly eaten foods.

Creamy Avocado Spinach Dip

It's hard to imagine what would make guacamole even more perfect than it already is. Enter spinach—a nutritional powerhouse and anti-inflammatory superstar that can happily join the party without interfering with the flavor. It's also kid-friendly, as evidenced by my two-year-old nephew who put his whole face in the bowl to lick it clean once he'd polished off the last of the dip. The kalamata olives are optional, but they add some nice saltiness that completely disguises the spinach.

Makes 6 servings

1 avocado

2 cups spinach

1 clove garlic, chopped

¼ cup olive oil, plus more as needed

2 tablespoons freshly squeezed lemon

1 teaspoon ground cumin

1 teaspoon sea salt

½ cup pitted kalamata olives (optional)

Scoop the avocado into a food processor. Add the spinach, garlic, and oil and blend. Additional oil can be added for a smoother texture. Add the lemon juice, cumin, and salt and blend until smooth. Add the olives and pulse until they are just chopped and incorporated.

Serve with assorted vegetables, such as carrots, cucumbers, cauliflower, or jicama. This dip also works great as a sandwich spread or a topping for bean and rice dishes.

Spinach contains high amounts of unique carotenoids, which are plant compounds that have been shown to calm inflammation, particularly in the digestive tract.

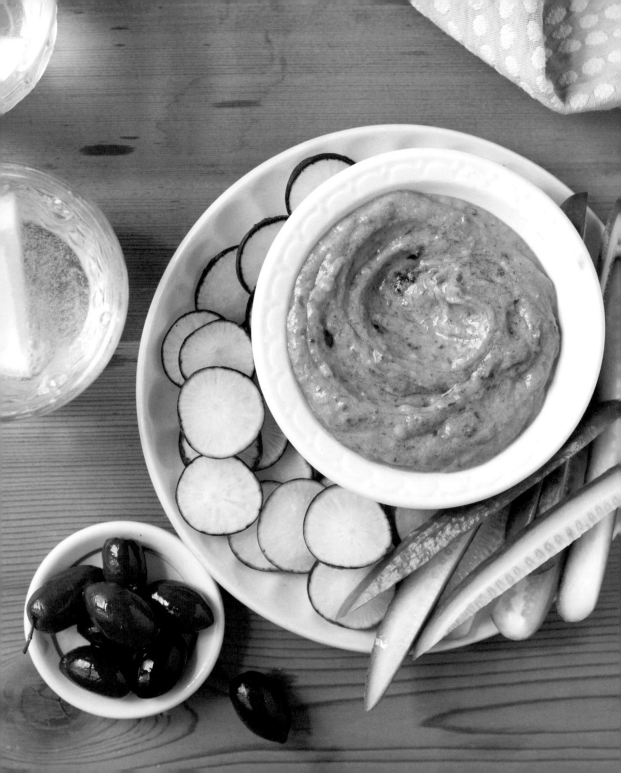

Artichoke and Basil Tapenade

Behold the beautiful olive! While technically a fruit, olives are better known for their fatty, salty, briny characteristics. They also happen to be one of the main components of a Mediterranean diet. I absolutely love the fact that we can get healthy fats and other anti-inflammatory compounds via such a remarkably tasty delivery system. The artichoke hearts add a different texture to the tapenade while the basil really helps balance the saltiness and elevates the flavor. I like to bring this snack to Super Bowl parties with the secret intention of unclogging the arteries of those who are overindulging in deep-fried chicken wings.

Makes 6 servings

1 (14-ounce) jar artichoke hearts marinated in olive oil
½ cup pitted green olives
½ cup pitted kalamata olives
4 to 5 large basil leaves or 2 teaspoons dried

Place all the ingredients in a blender or food processor and pulse until finely chopped but not pureed. Serve with assorted vegetables, such as carrots, cauliflower, or celery.

Tip: For a slightly fancier spin on this recipe, scoop the tapenade into endive leaves and arrange in a circular pattern on a large plate. This is a hit at parties, and it couldn't be easier for the host!

Anti-Inflammatory Trail Mix

Let's face it, trail mix has all the elements of a perfect snack. It's portable, it's satisfying, and it can be fun to eat. Unfortunately, the stuff available in the bulk section can be loaded with bits of candy, chocolate, and sugar-sweetened dried fruit. Sure, that might be what makes trail mix so much "fun," but if you have to mine out the candy and leave the nuts behind, you're really not doing yourself any favors. This homemade version is a delicious and nutritious solution. I encourage families to have a trail-mix-making party where you set out small bowls of nuts, seeds, and freeze-dried or unsweetened, unsulfured dried fruits, and have everyone create their own baggies of trail mix to take to school, work, or soccer practice.

Makes 16 (¼-cup) servings

1 cup raw almonds
1 cup shelled pistachios
1 cup shelled pumpkin seeds (pepitas)
½ cup freeze-dried blueberries
½ cup chopped unsweetened, unsulfured dried mangoes

1 cup Brazil nuts
1 cup macadamia nuts
1 cup sunflower seeds
1 cup unsweetened coconut flakes
½ cup raisins
½ cup dried figs
½ cup dried apricots

OPTIONAL ADDITIONS
1 cup walnuts
1 cup pecans

1 cup freeze-dried strawberries
1 cup freeze-dried raspberries

In a large bowl, combine the almonds, pistachios, pumpkin seeds, blueberries, and mangoes and toss well. Place any optional ingredients in small bowls and set them out to choose from. Combine a little of each desired item in a ¼-cup measuring cup and pour the contents from the cup into snack bags for preportioned, power-packed snacks that are ready to grab and go!

> Tip: Active adults and older children (8-plus years) may want to use ½ cup as a serving. Adults watching their weight and younger children should stick with the ¼-cup portion.

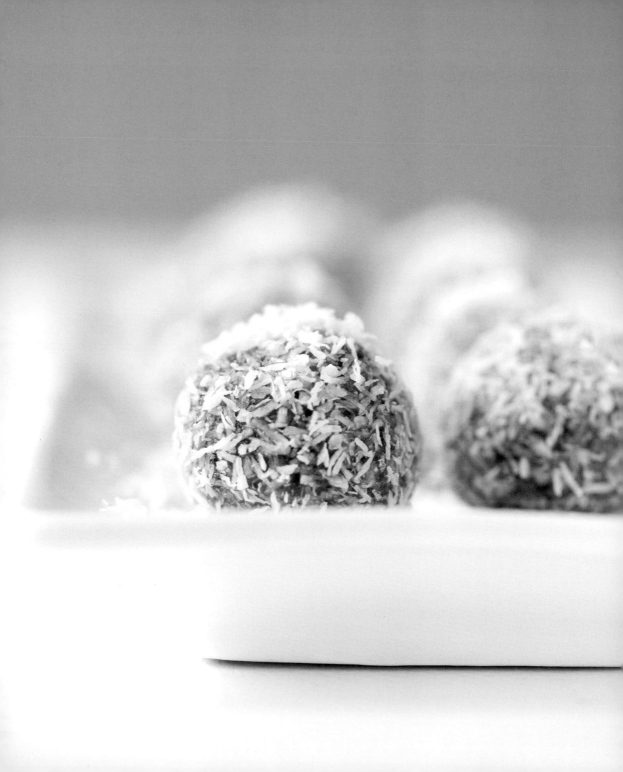

Nutty Coconut Energy Truffles

This recipe is definitely one of my top five greatest hits. The delectable combination of nuts, dried fruit, and coconut make it a universal favorite. I knew I was on to something when I took these yummy little treats to a campout with friends and they were gone within seconds of opening the container. My friends still talk about them today. They're a great high-energy snack to take along when hiking or biking, and they can be enjoyed as a much healthier stand-in for a candy bar. I recommend using Medjool dates because they're always fresh and moist with just the right amount of stickiness to bind these truffles together.

Makes 12 servings

2 cups raw walnuts
1 tablespoon ground cinnamon
⅛ teaspoon sea salt
½ cup pitted dates
½ cup dried cherries
2 tablespoons coconut oil

2 tablespoons almond butter
⅛ teaspoon almond extract
2 tablespoons maple syrup (optional)
½ cup unsweetened shredded coconut

Place the walnuts, cinnamon, and salt in a food processor. Process until the nuts are finely ground, about 1 minute. Add the dates, cherries, oil, almond butter, and extract. Process until well combined; the mixture should have a thick, sticky consistency. Check to see if you can form a truffle by rolling some of the mixture in your hands—if it falls apart easily, blend in the maple syrup.

Spread the coconut on a plate. Scoop the nut mixture with a large spoon and roll into 1-inch balls. Roll in the coconut until the balls are generously coated. Store the truffles in an airtight container in the refrigerator for up to 1 week and store extras in the freezer for up to 6 months.

Cinnamon inhibits the release of pro-inflammatory signals in the body and helps regulate blood sugar.

Tropical Quinoa Power Bars

Clients often ask me for ideas for portable, whole food snacks. While I think of quinoa as a super food, it's not generally known for portability. However, it's possible to take advantage of the sticky quality of freshly cooked quinoa, along with a few other key ingredients, to create a bar that travels well. I love the tropical trio of apricots, coconut, and macadamia nuts (which always seem like a treat!). I choose to go fairly light on the honey because I prefer a more subtle sweetness, but that can certainly be adjusted to taste.

Makes 12 servings

2 cups water
1 cup quinoa, rinsed and drained
¼ teaspoon sea salt
½ cup raw macadamia nuts
½ cup unsweetened shredded coconut

½ cup chopped dried apricots
2 tablespoons honey
2 tablespoons tahini
2 teaspoons ground cinnamon
¼ cup coconut flour

Place the water, quinoa, and salt in a medium saucepan over medium-high heat. Bring to a boil, cover, and reduce the heat to low. Simmer for 20 minutes without stirring. The quinoa will look like it sprouted and grew a tiny tail, and all of the water should be absorbed. Fluff with a fork and allow to cool for about 5 minutes.

In a large bowl, combine 2 cups of the quinoa (you'll have some leftover) with the macadamia nuts, coconut, and apricots. Stir in the honey, tahini, and cinnamon. Cover with the coconut flour and use your hands to knead everything together until well incorporated.

Shape the mixture into bars approximately 3 inches long and 1 inch thick. Place them in a shallow baking dish lined with parchment paper, cover, and refrigerate for 4 hours or overnight.

> Tip: I like to wrap these bars in parchment paper, then double wrap in foil, and store them in the freezer. I'll pull one out in the morning and toss it in my workbag, so I can look forward to a satisfying afternoon snack.

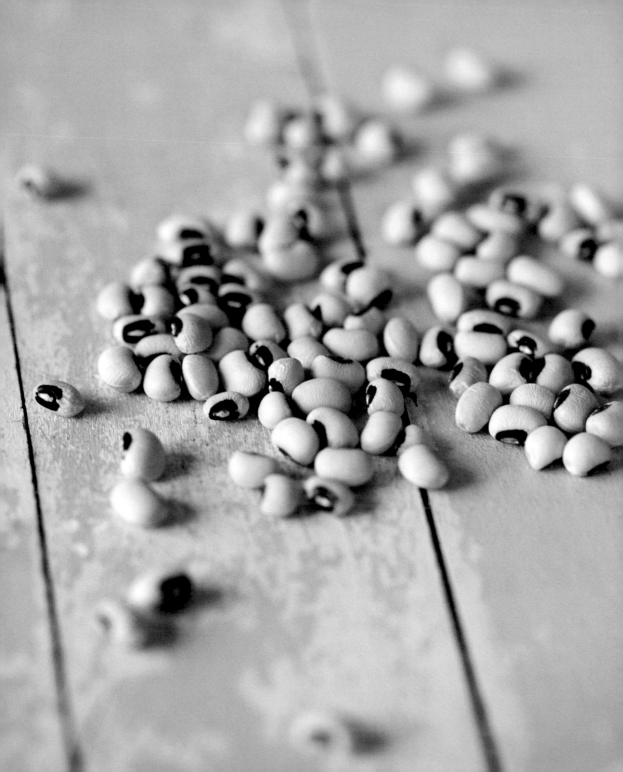

Soups and Stews

When I think of soups and stews, the first word that comes to mind is *nourishing*. A steaming bowl of soup can take the chill out of your bones and right wrongs of the world. In traditional Chinese medicine, soups are often described as tonics that have specific healing properties.

Many of the ingredients that are featured in this chapter have particular nutrients with known medicinal properties. So while these soups and stews are warming you up, they're cooling down systemic inflammation and strengthening your immune system.

Most of the recipes in this section make six to eight servings, so I recommend investing in some mason jars or glass storage containers and freezing a few servings for later. This helps prevent same-food fatigue, and you get to stock your freezer with some nourishing options for those nights that you just don't feel like cooking.

Mediterranean White Bean Soup

This Tuscan-inspired white bean soup is my go-to soup for clients who are just starting to practice anti-inflammatory eating. It's easy to make; contains beans and rice, which make a complete protein; and it freezes well, so leftovers can be spread out. I like to serve a small cup of this soup as a starter when I have a lamb dish on the menu, but it's definitely satisfying enough to be a meal all on its own.

Makes 8 servings

1 tablespoon extra-virgin olive oil
1 small red onion, chopped
1 medium green onion, chopped
1 cup sliced mushrooms
2 cloves garlic, minced
¼ cup dried Italian herbs
1 teaspoon sea salt, plus more for
   seasoning

2 quarts vegetable broth
1½ to 2 cups water
1 (15-ounce) can cannellini beans,
   rinsed and drained
¼ cup brown rice
3 cups chopped chard or spinach
Freshly ground black pepper

Heat the oil in a large stockpot over medium heat. Add the red and green onions and sauté until they start to sweat and become soft. Add the mushrooms, garlic, Italian herbs, and salt and cook, stirring occasionally, for 2 to 3 minutes, or until the mushrooms start to soften and release liquid.

Add the broth, water, beans, and rice; increase the heat to high; and bring the soup to a boil. Reduce the heat to medium-low and simmer for 45 minutes. Stir in the chard and continue simmering for another 10 to 15 minutes. Season to taste with salt and pepper and serve.

Roasted Cauliflower Soup with Gremolata

I created this soup for a cooking class on healthy hormone balance and was pleasantly surprised at how popular it was with the students. Roasting the cauliflower and leeks with turmeric and cumin really showcases their sweeter characteristics and makes the soup incredibly rich. As delicious as it tastes, the soup is lacking in color and tends to look pretty lonely in bowl without a colorful garnish. The gremolata adds a vibrant punch, and the parsley and lemon zest brighten up the flavor of the soup. If desired, you can use less broth to create more of a puree than a soup.

Makes 4 servings

1 leek (white and light green parts only), rinsed well and roughly chopped

1 large head cauliflower, separated into florets

2 tablespoons grapeseed oil

1 teaspoon ground turmeric

1 teaspoon ground cumin

1 teaspoon coarse sea salt

3 cups vegetable broth

½ cup coconut milk

FOR THE GREMOLATA:

½ cup finely chopped parsley

1 clove garlic, minced

1 tablespoon extra-virgin olive oil

1 teaspoon freshly grated lemon zest

Preheat the oven to 400 degrees F.

In a large bowl, toss the leek and cauliflower with the grapeseed oil, turmeric, and cumin. Spread on a baking pan, sprinkle with the salt, and roast for 15 to 20 minutes, or until the leeks start to brown.

Transfer the vegetables to a food processor. Add the broth and coconut milk and blend well, adding more broth or water as needed to achieve the desired consistency. Pour the soup into a saucepan and place over low heat until ready to serve.

To make the gremolata, combine the parsley, garlic, olive oil, and lemon zest in a small bowl and mix well.

Ladle the soup into bowls and top with a spoonful of gremolata.

Creamy Asparagus and Sunchoke Soup

When asparagus makes its debut at my local farmers' market, I know that spring has officially sprung. Time to trade in the winter squash and hearty root vegetables and make way for the lighter, greener foods that help us detox and recharge. Sunchokes, also known as Jerusalem artichokes, are rather unfortunate looking, but it's worth getting past their homely, knobby exterior. They have a slightly nutty, artichoke-like flavor that is subtle when combined with the stronger flavor of asparagus. They can also be shredded into a salad or roasted, so save a few for another day. You'll be pleasantly surprised at the creaminess of this soup without the use of any dairy products—the sunchokes and oats help smooth out the texture and give the illusion of a cream-based soup.

Makes 6 servings

1 tablespoon extra-virgin olive oil
1 leek (white and light green parts
    only), rinsed well and chopped
3 sunchokes, scrubbed and chopped
    into small pieces
1 bunch asparagus, ends trimmed,
    chopped into 1-inch pieces

1 quart mushroom broth
1 cup water
⅓ cup certified gluten-free rolled oats
1 teaspoon sea salt
½ teaspoon freshly ground black
    pepper

Drizzle the oil into a large saucepan or stockpot. Add the leek, stir until well coated with oil, and sauté over medium heat until soft. Add the sunchokes and asparagus and sauté for 2 to 3 minutes. Add the broth, water, oats, and salt. Bring to a boil over high heat, reduce the heat to medium-low, and simmer for 15 to 20 minutes.

Carefully transfer the soup in batches to a food processor and blend until smooth and creamy. Reheat on the stove top as needed and season with the pepper.

> Both asparagus and sunchokes contain inulin, an indigestible form of fiber that acts as a prebiotic and may help with inflammation in the gut.

Butternut Squash and White Bean Soup

Butternut squash soup must rank in the top three favorite soups among adults and kids alike. I'd always found it to be a bit too sweet for my liking, which is why I decided to cut some of the sweetness by adding white beans. And then of course the nutritionist side of me loves the fact that adding beans really increases the fiber, adds essential minerals, and makes the soup heartier and more satiating. Now I'm proud to report that I, too, am a butternut squash soup lover! For dinner parties, this soup is fun to serve in hollowed-out gourds or mini pumpkins. It's festive and looks beautiful on the table.

Makes 6 servings

1 tablespoon extra-virgin olive oil
1 small yellow onion, chopped
1 medium butternut squash, peeled, seeded, and cubed
2 cloves garlic, minced
6 cups vegetable broth
1 (15-ounce) can cannellini or other white beans, rinsed and drained

2 teaspoons sea salt
1 teaspoon ground cumin
½ teaspoon ground coriander
¼ teaspoon cayenne pepper
1 teaspoon freshly ground black pepper

Drizzle the oil into a large saucepan and add the onions, stirring until well coated with oil. Sauté over medium heat until the onions soften and start to become translucent, about 3 to 4 minutes. Add the squash, garlic, broth, beans, salt, cumin, coriander, and cayenne and bring to a boil. Reduce the heat to low, cover, and simmer for 35 to 40 minutes.

Carefully transfer small batches of the soup to a food processor or blender, blend until smooth, and then return to the pan to keep warm. Season with the pepper.

> Tip: This soup can be stored in an airtight container in the refrigerator for 4 to 5 days and also freezes well. With leftovers, I like to add fresh spinach or chopped kale and serve it over quinoa, just to change it up.

Slow-Cooked Black Bean and Broccoli Stew

Finding good vegetarian slow cooker recipes can be challenging, which is what inspired this creation. Black beans tend to require a longer cooking time than most beans, so they're perfectly suited for slow cooking. The blend of herbs and spices gives this stew a Moroccan feel and creates a heavenly aroma that will welcome you home after a long day of work. If you want another shortcut, you can look for a North African spice blend called ras el hanout. It has many of the same anti-inflammatory spices called for here (plus a few extras!). I usually make some red rice or quinoa for serving during the stew's last half hour of cooking.

Makes 6 servings

1 cup dried black beans, soaked overnight
4 cups water
1 small white onion, diced
1 teaspoon ground black mustard seed
1 teaspoon garlic powder
1 teaspoon ground cumin
1 teaspoon ground turmeric

1 teaspoon ground fennel seed
1 teaspoon chili powder
½ teaspoon ground coriander
¼ teaspoon ground cinnamon
¼ teaspoon ground ginger
2 teaspoons sea salt
1 head broccoli, separated into florets
Rice or quinoa, for serving

Rinse and drain the beans and put them in a slow cooker with the water, onion, and all of the spices except for salt. Cover and cook on low for 8 hours.

Add the salt and broccoli, cover, and cook for another 30 minutes. Serve over rice or quinoa.

Phytonutrients in broccoli have been found to suppress the inflammatory signaling system and may also decrease allergic responses that lead to inflammation.

Three-Bean Stew with Red Quinoa

This vegetarian stew has a colorful array of beans and features the lesser-known adzuki bean, a small red bean that's a particular favorite in macrobiotic diets. It's a nutritional powerhouse, loaded with minerals and easier to digest than some other beans. Kombu is a sea vegetable (aka seaweed) that helps tenderize the beans and imparts minerals during cooking. I like to think of it as the bay leaf for beans. Adding chunky vegetables and quinoa to this stew gives it a hearty enough texture to satisfy any meat-eating friends or family. Note that the black beans should be soaked separately as they are cooked longer than the others.

Makes 6 servings

⅓ cup dried black beans, soaked overnight
⅓ cup dried adzuki beans, soaked overnight
⅓ cup dried cannellini beans, soaked overnight
3 cups vegetable broth
1 (6-inch) strip kombu
1 tablespoon coconut oil
1 small yellow onion, diced
2 small zucchini, chopped
1 unpeeled sweet potato, scrubbed and chopped into ½-inch cubes

2 cloves garlic, minced
¼ cup red quinoa
1 tablespoon chili powder
2 teaspoons ground cumin
1 teaspoon ground ginger
1 teaspoon sea salt
½ teaspoon ground cinnamon

OPTIONAL ADDITIONS
1 cup corn kernels
¼ cup diced green chilies
1 cup fire-roasted peppers

Rinse the beans thoroughly and drain. Put the black beans in a large stockpot with the broth and kombu. Bring to a boil over medium-high heat, then reduce the heat to medium-low and simmer for 20 minutes. Add the adzuki and cannellini beans and simmer for another 60 to 90 minutes, or until all the beans are tender.

Meanwhile, heat the oil in a medium sauté pan over medium heat. Add the onion and sauté until translucent. Add the zucchini and sauté for 3 to 4 minutes. Set aside.

When the beans are tender, discard the kombu. Add the onions and zucchini, sweet potato, garlic, quinoa, chili powder, cumin, ginger, salt, and cinnamon to the stockpot. Stir in any optional items at this time. Reduce the heat to low and simmer for 30 to 40 minutes to allow the flavors to mingle and the sweet potato to soften.

Quinoa is higher in healthy unsaturated fats than most other grains and even contains a small amount of omega-3s. It's also loaded with a unique blend of phytonutrients known to be anti-inflammatory.

Caramelized Carrot and Ginger Soup

Carrots are a great example of a vegetable with multiple personalities. As a child, I would only eat them raw, straight out of my grandmother's garden. I had no use for peeled carrots in general, and I detested cooked ones (thankfully I'm over that now). Roasted carrots, slightly caramelized with a little bit of sweetener, are an entirely different experience than steamed or sautéed carrots. The buttery sweetness of the caramelized carrots makes this recipe unique compared to other carrot-ginger soups. Coconut palm sugar is great here because it's a low-glycemic sweetener that is reminiscent of brown sugar.

Makes 6 servings

8 unpeeled carrots, scrubbed well and cut into 1-inch chunks
1 small yellow onion, sliced into thick rings
1 tablespoon coconut oil, melted
2 tablespoons coconut palm sugar
2 cups vegetable broth
½ cup water
1½ teaspoons freshly grated peeled ginger
½ teaspoon sea salt

Preheat the oven to 400 degrees F.

Place the carrots and onion in a large bowl and toss with the coconut oil and palm sugar until well coated. Spread the vegetables evenly on a baking pan. Roast in the oven for 30 minutes, or until the onions start to caramelize and the carrots begin to turn golden brown.

Transfer the vegetables to a food processor. Add the broth, water, ginger, and salt and blend until smooth. Reheat the soup in a saucepan over medium heat and serve warm.

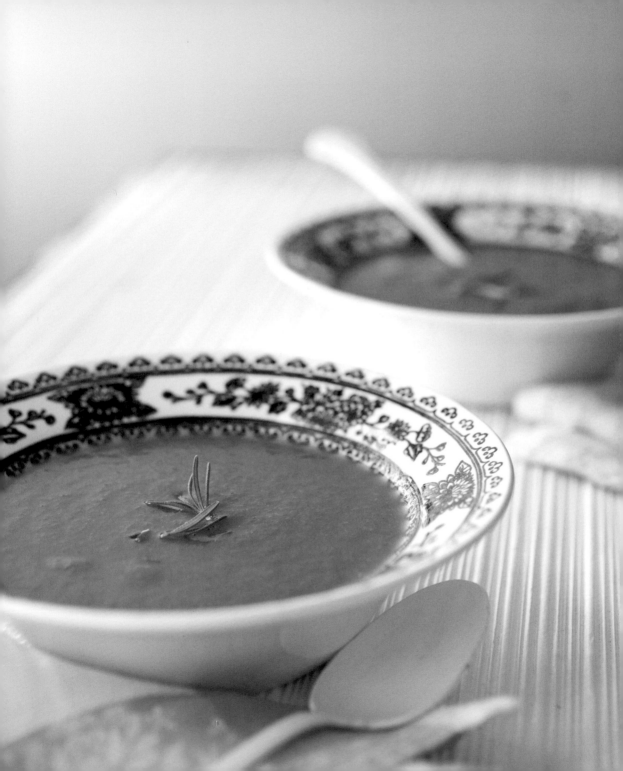

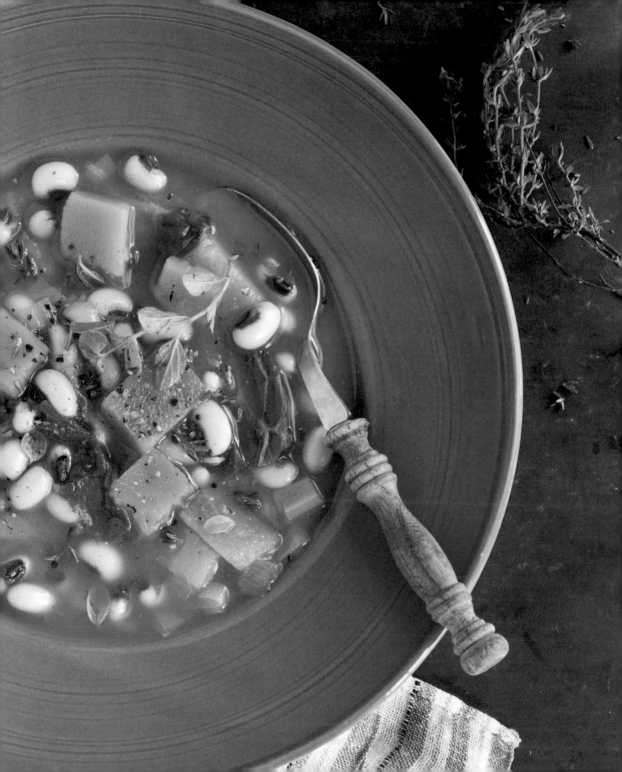

Black-Eyed Pea and Escarole Soup

I remember the first time I saw someone add escarole to soup, I thought to myself, "Why is that person putting leaf lettuce into soup?" As I learned when I tasted the soup, escarole is perfectly suited for light cooking and is an extremely versatile leafy green. It has a slightly bitter note that mellows when cooked, and it's perfectly balanced in this recipe by the sweetness from the butternut squash. Save yourself some time and head to the frozen foods section to find squash that's already cubed and ready to use.

Makes 6 servings

1½ cups dried black-eyed peas, soaked overnight
6 cups vegetable broth
2 cloves garlic, minced
1 tablespoon fresh thyme or 2 teaspoons dried
1 tablespoon fresh oregano or 2 teaspoons dried
1 tablespoon coconut oil

1 large or 2 small leeks (white and light green parts only), rinsed well and sliced into half moons
2 stalks celery, chopped
1 cup frozen cubed butternut squash
1 head escarole, coarsely chopped (about 2 cups)
1 teaspoon sea salt
½ teaspoon freshly ground black pepper

Rinse and drain the black-eyed peas and put in a large stockpot. Add the broth, garlic, thyme, and oregano. Bring to a boil, and then reduce the heat to medium-low to maintain a simmer.

Meanwhile, heat the oil in a medium skillet over medium heat. Add the leeks and celery and sauté for 5 minutes, or until the leeks sweat and the celery starts to soften. Transfer the vegetables to the stockpot, cover, and simmer for 40 minutes.

Stir the squash and escarole into the soup and simmer for another 20 minutes. Season with the salt and pepper and serve. Leftovers can be stored in the freezer for up to 6 months.

> Escarole is a good source of vitamin K, which is an important nutrient that helps regulate the body's inflammatory processes. One cup provides more than 100 percent of the recommended daily intake.

Lentil and Spinach Stew with Roasted Garlic

Lentils are so delightfully simple. There's no soaking required, and the cooking time is shorter than most legumes. Red lentils are often the first choice for dal, an Indian dish that's the consistency of mashed potatoes. This is primarily because red lentils don't hold their shape when you cook them, which makes them desirable for thicker soups and stews. In this recipe, you'll be simmering them for ninety minutes over low heat so they will soften and break apart, blending into the stew. The addition of balsamic vinegar and roasted garlic really brings the flavors together and makes this the ultimate anti-inflammatory comfort food!

Makes 6 servings

1 head garlic
1 tablespoon extra-virgin olive oil, divided
2 leeks (white and light green parts only), rinsed well and sliced into half moons
1 carrot, diced
1 stalk celery, diced
3 cups vegetable broth
1½ cups water

1½ cups dried red lentils, rinsed and drained
2 bay leaves
1 tablespoon fresh thyme or 2 teaspoons dried
1½ cups chopped spinach
3 tablespoons balsamic vinegar
1 teaspoon sea salt
Freshly ground black pepper (or crushed red pepper flakes for more heat)

Preheat the oven to 350 degrees F.

Slice the top off the head of garlic to expose the cloves. Drizzle with 1 teaspoon of the oil and wrap the head in foil. Place in the oven and roast for 50 minutes.

Meanwhile, heat the remaining 2 teaspoons oil in a large saucepan or stockpot over medium heat. Add the leeks, carrot, and celery and sauté for 5 minutes, or until the leeks begin to sweat and the carrots and celery soften. Add the broth, water, lentils, bay leaves, and thyme. Reduce the heat to low and simmer, stirring occasionally, for 50 to 60 minutes.

Discard the bay leaves. Gently squeeze the roasted garlic cloves into the stew. Stir in the spinach and balsamic vinegar. Season with the salt and pepper and serve.

Vegetable and Chicken Pho

When pho mania hit Seattle, I was late to the party. I'm not sure what the holdup was, because pho has all of my prerequisites for the perfect comfort food. It's warm, it has noodles, and the aroma just feels like coming home. After making up for lost time with countless pho outings, I decided to try to create a slow cooker version with less meat, more veggies, and plenty of flavor. If you can't find Kaffir lime leaves, just substitute a teaspoon of lime zest and a generous squeeze of lime juice. When serving the pho, choose a selection of suggested toppings from the list to pass at the table.

Makes 6 servings

1 (8-ounce) bone-in free-range organic chicken breast, skin removed
3 green onions, chopped
5 cloves garlic
1 tablespoon chopped peeled fresh ginger
1 ounce dried porcini mushrooms
1 quart mushroom broth
1 quart water
2 tablespoons Coconut Aminos (tamari or Bragg Liquid Aminos if avoiding soy)
2 tablespoons agave nectar
2 tablespoons five-spice powder
2 teaspoons sea salt
4 ounces wide rice noodles
1 cup chopped bok choy
1 cup chopped broccoli florets
5 Kaffir lime leaves

FOR SERVING:
1 cup bean sprouts
1 cup shredded carrots
1 cup chopped fresh basil leaves
1 cup chopped fresh cilantro
Sriracha, hot peppers, or crushed red pepper flakes

Place the chicken in a slow cooker. Add the green onions, garlic, ginger, porcinis, broth, water, aminos, agave, five-spice powder, and salt. Cover and cook on low for 8 hours.

Remove the chicken and use a fork to shred the meat from the bone. Return the shredded chicken to the slow cooker. Add the noodles, bok choy, broccoli, and lime leaves. Add more water to cover as needed. Cover, increase the temperature to high, and cook for an additional 30 minutes. Discard the lime leaves.

Ladle the soup into bowls and offer the desired selection of ingredients for serving on the side.

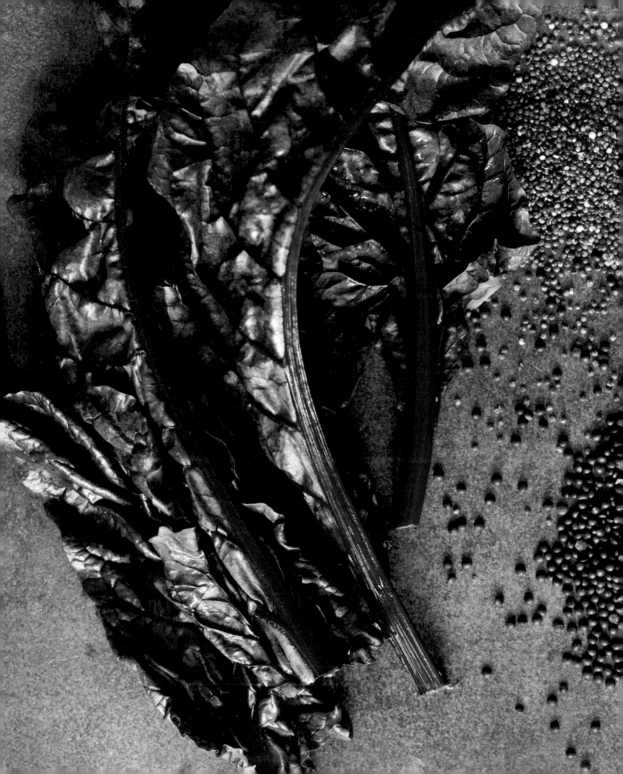

Salads and Sides

The goal of an anti-inflammatory Mediterranean-style diet is to make sure that vegetables occupy at least half of the real estate on your plate. If that feels like a substantial shift from what your plate looks like now, please don't panic. This chapter of salads and sides is designed to make veggie eating second nature.

There are a wide variety of vegetables featured in the recipes that follow, and some may be outside of your usual repertoire. Challenge yourself to be an explorer. Why limit yourself to romaine lettuce and carrots when you can tantalize your taste buds with fennel, kohlrabi, and chard? If you look beyond your usual produce picks and expand your vegetable horizon, you'll exponentially increase the variety of anti-inflammatory nutrients in your diet, and what's more, you'll actually enjoy it!

Remember that nightshades (tomatoes, potatoes, peppers, and eggplant) are not featured in these recipes to accommodate those who might have an inflammatory reaction to those foods. However, if you are not one of those people, I encourage you to add them for more color, flavor, and phytonutrients.

Wilted Kale Salad with Shredded Beets and Carrots

This salad gives you all the benefits that raw kale, beets, and carrots have to offer. No nutrients were destroyed in the making of this dish. You'll wilt the kale with the heat of your own hands when you thoroughly massage the dressing into the leaves. This is a great way to break down kale and make it more tender and enjoyable to eat raw. And you get the added benefit of silky smooth hands from the avocado and olive oil.

Makes 6 servings

2 bunches kale, stemmed and coarsely
   chopped
1 avocado
2 tablespoons balsamic vinegar
1 tablespoon extra-virgin olive oil

½ teaspoon sea salt
4 carrots, shredded
2 unpeeled beets, scrubbed and
   shredded
¼ cup pine nuts, toasted

Put the kale in a large bowl. Scoop the avocado into the bowl and drizzle with the balsamic vinegar, oil, and salt. Using both hands, massage the avocado and dressing into the kale. It will start to take on a wilted appearance as it gets tender.

Add the carrots, beets, and pine nuts. Toss well and serve.

Beets contain phytonutrients that support healthy detoxification and reduce inflammation in the body.

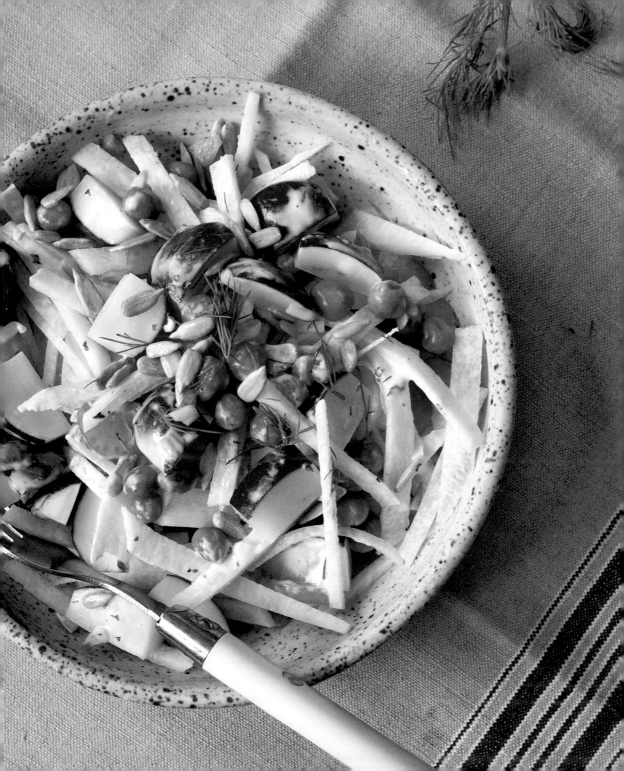

Spring Pea and Jicama Salad

There's a relatively short window of opportunity to get your hands on some fresh spring peas, but it's a window you don't want to miss. When you open the pod and see the vibrant, perfect green row of plump little peas, you'll know right away that you're in for a treat. Don't fret if you miss the spring pea harvest—frozen peas are a perfectly suitable option. This light and creamy salad will dress up any barbecue or picnic. The firm yet creamy texture of the peas is offset by the crunch from the jicama and celery. A tangy lemon-dill dressing brings this beautifully balanced salad together.

Makes 6 servings

1½ cups shelled spring peas, or 1 (10-ounce) bag frozen petite peas, thawed
10 radishes, quartered
2 stalks celery, chopped
1 small jicama, peeled and shredded
¼ cup sunflower seeds
½ cup Soy-Free Vegenaise

2 tablespoons freshly squeezed lemon juice
1 tablespoon apple cider vinegar
1 clove garlic, minced
1 teaspoon dried dill
1 teaspoon dried basil
1 teaspoon sea salt

In a large bowl, combine the peas, radishes, celery, jicama, and sunflower seeds.

In a small bowl, whisk together the Vegenaise, lemon juice, vinegar, garlic, dill, basil, and salt.

Drizzle the dressing over the salad and toss until all ingredients are well coated.

Rainbow Quinoa with Roasted Asparagus and Adzuki Beans

This colorful bean and grain salad is packed with nutrients and makes a great side dish or a tasty stand-alone lunch. Quinoa is one of the most nutritious whole grains, and adzuki beans outshine many other beans because of their mineral content. If you can't find rainbow quinoa, traditional or red quinoa will work just fine. You can play with variations of this recipe by substituting different beans (such as black, chickpea, or pinto) and switch up the veggies based on what's in season.

Makes 4 servings

1 pound asparagus, ends trimmed, cut into 1-inch pieces
6 tablespoons extra-virgin olive oil, divided
2 cups vegetable broth
1 cup rainbow quinoa
2 cups stemmed and chopped chard
1 (15-ounce) can adzuki beans, rinsed and drained
½ cup chopped kalamata olives
2 tablespoons freshly squeezed lime juice
1 teaspoon agave nectar or honey
1 teaspoon sea salt
Freshly ground black pepper

Preheat the oven to 375 degrees F.

In a large bowl, toss the asparagus with 2 tablespoons of the oil. Spread the asparagus on a baking pan and roast for 15 to 20 minutes, or until tender.

Meanwhile, in a large saucepan over high heat, combine the broth and quinoa. Bring to a boil, reduce the heat to low, cover, and simmer for 20 minutes without stirring. Measure 1 cup of the quinoa to use in the salad, reserving the extra for another use.

In a large bowl, combine the asparagus, 1 cup quinoa, chard, beans, and olives.

In a small bowl, whisk together the remaining ¼ cup oil, lime juice, and agave. Drizzle over the salad and toss until well coated. Season with the salt and pepper and serve.

Wild Rice and Roasted Vegetables

This dish is a mainstay in my repertoire of sides because it's simple, versatile, and a crowd-pleaser. The types of veggies I roast correspond with what's in season, so sometimes it includes more root vegetables, like rutabaga, turnips, and beets, and other times it includes zucchini, mushrooms, and sweet potatoes. Regardless of the combination I use, dinner guests almost always ask for the recipe.

Makes 6 servings

2 cups vegetable or mushroom broth
1 cup wild rice, rinsed well and drained
3 medium carrots, chopped into 1-inch chunks
1 zucchini, chopped into 1-inch chunks
1 small yellow onion, chopped
2 cups broccoli florets
1½ cups cremini mushrooms, quartered

2 tablespoons grapeseed or sunflower oil
1½ teaspoons coarse sea salt, divided
3 tablespoons extra-virgin olive oil
2 tablespoons balsamic vinegar
2 cloves garlic, minced
1 tablespoon dried Italian herbs

Preheat the oven to 425 degrees F.

Put the broth and rice in a large saucepan and bring to a boil over high heat. Reduce the heat to low, cover, and simmer for approximately 50 minutes, or until the broth is absorbed and the rice is tender but not mushy.

Meanwhile, combine the carrots, zucchini, onion, broccoli, and mushrooms in a large bowl. Drizzle with the grapeseed oil, sprinkle with 1 teaspoon of the salt, and toss until well coated.

Spread the vegetables in a single layer on a large baking pan. Roast for 20 minutes, stirring after 10 minutes. Transfer the vegetables back to the large bowl. Stir in the rice.

In a small bowl, whisk together the olive oil, balsamic vinegar, garlic, remaining ½ teaspoon salt, and Italian herbs. Drizzle over the vegetables and rice and toss until well combined.

Brussels Sprout Slaw

Eating brussels sprouts raw may seem like absolute madness to most. Until you think about the fact that it's just baby cabbage, so it's actually genius to use it for slaw. If you object to mayonnaise-laden salads, this will be a welcome replacement. The sprouts and purple cabbage are nicely dressed in a light vinaigrette with a bit of an Asian flair. The sesame oil offsets the grassy notes of the flaxseed oil and balances perfectly with the tangy sweet rice wine vinegar. I use flaxseed oil because it's a good vegetarian source of omega-3s, but you can substitute extra-virgin olive oil if you don't have flaxseed on hand.

Makes 6 servings

3 tablespoons rice wine vinegar
2 tablespoons toasted sesame oil
1 tablespoon flaxseed oil
1 tablespoon agave nectar
½ pound brussels sprouts, ends trimmed

½ small head purple cabbage
¼ cup golden raisins
2 teaspoons poppy seeds

In a small bowl, whisk together the rice wine vinegar, sesame oil, flaxseed oil, and agave. Set aside.

Chop the brussels sprouts into fine strips or use a food processor to shred them. Chop the purple cabbage into thin strips or shred in a food processor.

Combine the brussels sprouts and cabbage in a large bowl with the raisins and poppy seeds. Drizzle the vinaigrette over the slaw and toss thoroughly to coat.

> Tip: This slaw gets better after marinating in the dressing for at least a couple hours in the refrigerator. I love to pair leftovers with grilled halibut or cod for fish tacos.

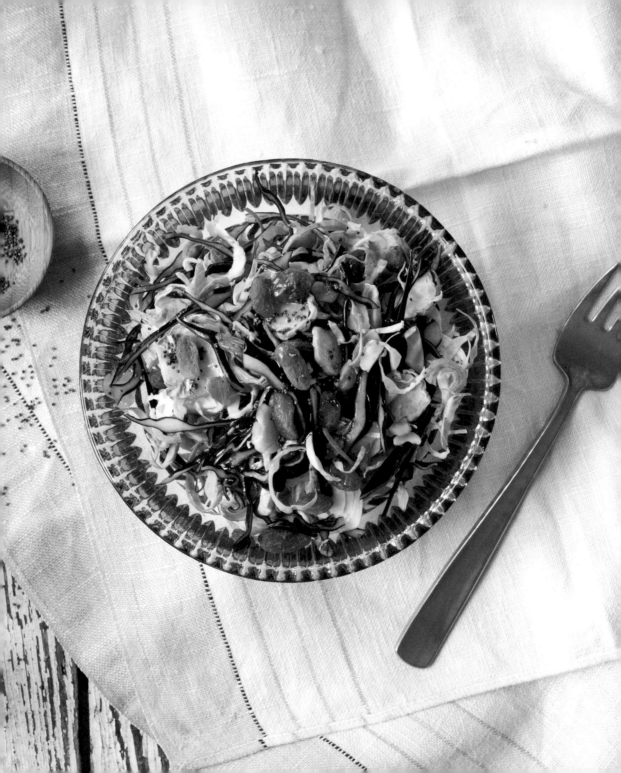

Bhutanese Rice and Flageolet Bean Salad

If you've ever been served red rice when you ordered brown at a Thai restaurant, chances are it was Bhutanese rice. This nutty, earthy, red-toned rice is as nutritious as brown rice but cooks in half the time and is a whole lot more interesting. Flageolet beans are a favorite in French cuisine, and their pale green hue makes them a beautiful companion to the red rice. If you can't find flageolets, you can substitute cannellini beans or baby limas. Kombu is a type of seaweed that imparts minerals and helps break down the fiber in the beans.

Makes 6 servings

1 cup dried flageolet beans, soaked overnight
3 cups water
1 (6-inch) strip kombu (optional)
1 cup Bhutanese red rice
1½ cups vegetable broth
1 bunch chard, stemmed and chopped

1 small fennel bulb, chopped
½ cup chopped fresh parsley
½ cup sunflower seeds
¼ cup extra-virgin olive oil
2 tablespoons sherry vinegar
1 clove garlic, minced
¼ teaspoon sea salt

Rinse and drain the beans and transfer to a large saucepan. Add the water and kombu and bring to a boil over high heat. Reduce the heat to low and simmer, uncovered, for 45 to 50 minutes, or until the beans are tender. Discard the kombu and drain any excess water from the beans. Measure 1 cup of the beans for use in the salad, reserving any extra for another use.

Meanwhile, combine the rice and broth in a medium saucepan and bring to a boil over high heat. Cover, reduce the heat to low, and simmer for 20 minutes. Measure 1 cup of the rice for use in the salad, reserving any extra for another use.

In a large bowl, combine the 1 cup beans, 1 cup rice, chard, fennel, parsley, and sunflower seeds.

In a small bowl, whisk together the oil, vinegar, garlic, and salt. Drizzle over the salad and toss until well coated. Serve warm or cold.

Warm Brussels Sprout Salad with Pecans and Currants

I have converted more brussels sprout haters with this recipe than any other. Sautéing the shredded sprouts gives them an almost creamy texture. Adding the toasted pecans and currants brings in just enough sweetness to disguise any lingering bitterness from the sprouts. I've used this as a side dish for Thanksgiving meals, and it pairs very well with poultry or white fish.

Makes 6 servings

½ cup pecans
2 tablespoons extra-virgin olive oil
1 pound brussels sprouts, ends
    trimmed, thinly sliced

¼ cup dried currants
1 teaspoon sea salt
¼ cup vegetable broth

Preheat the oven to 350 degrees F.

Spread the pecans on a baking pan and roast for 8 to 10 minutes, or until fragrant. Transfer to a food processor and pulse until roughly chopped. (Alternatively, you can coarsely chop the pecans by hand.) Set aside.

In a large sauté pan or cast-iron skillet, heat the oil over medium heat. Add the brussels sprouts and toss until thoroughly coated with oil. Add the currants and salt and sauté, stirring occasionally for 2 to 3 minutes. Deglaze the pan with the broth, scraping up any brown bits. Reduce the heat to medium-low, cover, and simmer for 10 to 15 minutes, until the brussels sprouts are tender. Remove from the heat, stir in the pecans, and serve.

> Brussels sprouts help reduce inflammation in a number of ways. Compounds in this member of the cabbage family help the body process toxins, fight off free radicals, and block pro-inflammatory pathways.

Kale and Kohlrabi Salad with Creamy Avocado Vinaigrette

I like to dress up a classic kale salad with some interesting shredded veggies. Kohlrabi is one of the lesser-known members of the cabbage family and often gets neglected because of its unusual appearance. It has the texture of a turnip but tastes more like a cross between a radish and cauliflower. The avocado-based dressing mimics a creamy balsamic vinaigrette, and it makes this kale salad (or any salad!) irresistible. This salad will hold up for a couple days in the refrigerator, and the flavor and texture get even better with time.

Makes 4 servings

1 small bunch kale, stemmed and finely shredded
2 small or 1 medium kohlrabi, peeled and shredded
2 carrots, shredded
1 avocado

3 tablespoons balsamic vinegar
2 tablespoons extra-virgin olive oil
½ teaspoon sea salt, plus more for seasoning
1 cup water
¼ cup hemp or sunflower seeds

Combine the kale, kohlrabi, and carrots in a large bowl and toss well.

Scoop the avocado into a food processor or blender along with the balsamic vinegar, oil, and salt. With the machine running, slowly add the water.

Drizzle the dressing over the salad, add the sunflower seeds, and toss until all ingredients are well coated. Season to taste with salt.

Kale easily tops the list of anti-inflammatory vegetables. It's a good source of omega-3s, and it's rich in vitamin K, which is an inflammation regulator.

Oven-Roasted Beets with Sautéed Greens

Whenever I encounter someone who claims to dislike beets, I always ask whether they've ever tried them roasted. It's such a different experience than eating them canned or steamed beyond recognition. Oven-roasted beets have an earthy sweetness that I find irresistible. And not only are the beet greens loaded with vitamin K, an anti-inflammatory nutrient, they are also delicious when lightly sautéed. Early-season beets often have greens that are delicate enough to use raw in a salad. However, in the winter, when the greens are heartier, I prefer to sauté them or add them to soups.

Makes 4 servings

3 medium red or gold beets with greens attached	1 tablespoon coarse sea or kosher salt
2 tablespoons grapeseed or sunflower oil	2 teaspoons extra-virgin olive oil
	1 tablespoon balsamic vinegar

Preheat the oven to 375 degrees F.

Trim the beet greens from the beets and set aside. Thoroughly scrub the unpeeled beets and trim off any stems or roots. Chop the beets into 1-inch chunks and toss with the grapeseed oil until well coated. Spread the beets on a baking pan, sprinkle with the salt, and roast for about 25 minutes, or until the beets are tender.

Meanwhile, wash the beet greens thoroughly, trim the stems, and cut the leaves into thin strips. Heat the olive oil in a large sauté pan over medium heat, add the greens, and sauté until wilted, 3 to 4 minutes.

Toss the beets and greens in a large bowl with the balsamic vinegar and serve.

> Many of the unique phytonutrients in beets have anti-inflammatory effects. The mechanism of action is similar to some of the nonsteroidal anti-inflammatory drugs but without the side effects!

Braised Greens and Roasted Fennel with Silky Walnut Sauce

Covering half your plate with braised greens is one of the best ways to start building an anti-inflammatory plate. Braising, which really just means sautéing in oil and then steaming with liquid, is a quick and easy way to soften up hearty greens. And just to make it even *more* interesting, roasted fennel joins the party to share its sweet anise flavor and its own unique anti-inflammatory benefits. You'll top it all off with a silky, savory walnut sauce that not only makes the greens irresistibly delicious, but it also gives you an extra boost of omega-3s. Roasting the walnuts and adding a touch of maple syrup help to mellow any lingering bitterness of the greens.

Makes 4 servings

FOR THE WALNUT SAUCE:
1 cup raw walnuts
½ cup canned butter beans, rinsed
    and drained
1 tablespoon tahini
1 tablespoon maple syrup
1 teaspoon sea salt
¾ cup water

2 fennel bulbs, cut into 1-inch chunks
2 teaspoons grapeseed oil
½ teaspoon coarse sea or kosher salt
2 tablespoons extra-virgin olive oil
1 shallot, diced
1 cup sliced shiitake mushrooms
1 bunch kale or chard, stemmed and
    cut into ribbons
2 tablespoons mirin
1 tablespoon balsamic vinegar

Preheat the oven to 350 degrees F.

To make the walnut sauce, first spread the walnuts on a baking pan and roast for 10 minutes. Allow to cool slightly, then transfer to a food processor along with the beans, tahini, maple syrup, and salt. With the machine running, slowly add the water until the mixture is thin enough to drizzle. Set aside.

Increase the oven temperature to 400 degrees F.

In a medium bowl, toss the fennel and grapeseed oil to coat. Spread the fennel on a baking pan, sprinkle with the salt, and roast for 40 minutes.

Put the olive oil and shallots in a large sauté pan over medium heat and cook for 2 minutes. Add the mushrooms and sauté for 5 minutes. Add the kale and sauté until it begins to wilt. Add the fennel to the pan along with the mirin and balsamic vinegar. Reduce the heat to low, cover, and simmer for 5 minutes.

To serve, divide the braised vegetables among four plates and drizzle each with the walnut sauce.

Tip: The Silky Walnut Sauce also works well as a creamy salad dressing. You can even drizzle it over fresh baked pears or apples for a delectable sweet and savory dessert.

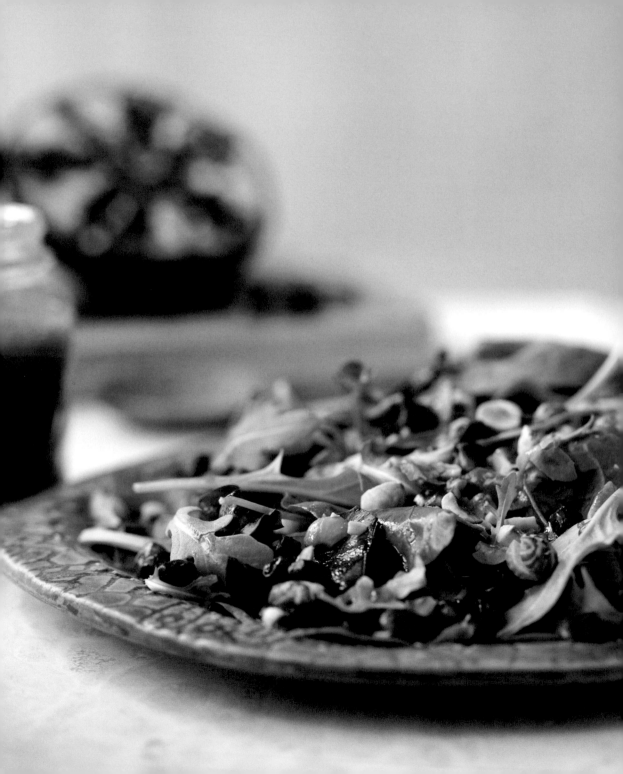

Super Greens Salad with Pomegranate and Toasted Hazelnuts

I was tempted to call this the Ultimate Antioxidant Salad, but it just didn't seem quite as sexy. All of the featured ingredients are loaded with immune-boosting, cancer-fighting, heart-protecting antioxidants. But that's not the best part. The wooden-spoon method of getting the seeds out of the pomegranate is a great stress reliever and just downright fun. I taught this technique to a friend's two young sons at a Thanksgiving gathering, and they're still talking about it (and they now *love* pomegranates).

Makes 6 servings

¾ cup raw hazelnuts	¼ teaspoon sea salt
1 pomegranate	2 cups spinach
¼ cup extra-virgin olive oil	1 cup arugula
1 tablespoon champagne vinegar	1 cup stemmed and chopped chard
1 teaspoon honey	

Preheat the oven to 350 degrees F.

Spread the hazelnuts on a baking pan and roast for 10 minutes. Transfer the nuts to a clean dish towel while they're still warm. Wrap the pile of nuts in the towel and aggressively massage them to remove the skins. Coarsely chop the hazelnuts and set aside.

Cut the pomegranate in half. Over a medium bowl, hold one half of the pomegranate, cut side down. Use a wooden spoon to repeatedly strike the sides of the pomegranate while gently squeezing with the hand holding it. Seeds will start to fall into the bowl. If no seeds are falling, put some muscle into it. Empty the seeds from both halves of the pomegranate into the bowl and pick out any of the white membrane that may have also fallen in. Pour the seeds through a strainer over a small bowl to capture the pomegranate juice. Measure ½ cup of the pomegranate seeds to use in the salad, reserving any extras for another use.

continued

Add the oil to the pomegranate juice and whisk in the vinegar, honey, and salt until well blended.

In a large bowl, combine the spinach, arugula, and chard. Add the hazelnuts and ½ cup pomegranate seeds. Drizzle the dressing over the salad and toss until the greens are well coated.

> Antioxidants help destroy free radicals in the body and prevent oxidation, both of which can cause inflammation. They also help support the immune system.

Shredded Cabbage and Snow Pea Sauté

I have such an appreciation for vegetarian Indian dishes that bring vegetables to life with interesting combinations of herbs and spices. That's what makes this recipe one of my all-time favorite anti-inflammatory side dishes. Heating the mustard seeds, turmeric, and asafetida in oil unlocks the powerful flavors that welcome the cabbage and snow peas with open arms. Asafetida is an extremely pungent spice (with some unflattering nicknames) that is used almost exclusively in Indian cuisine. It's commonly used in curry and dal and is thought of as a replacement for onions or garlic. A little bit goes a long way!

Makes 4 servings

2 teaspoons black mustard seeds
1 teaspoon coarse sea salt
½ teaspoon ground turmeric
¼ teaspoon asafetida
2 tablespoons coconut oil

½ large head green cabbage, shredded (about 2 cups)
1 cup snow peas
¼ cup water

In a small bowl, combine the mustard seeds, salt, turmeric, and asafetida.

Heat the oil in a cast-iron skillet or large sauté pan over medium-high heat. Add the spices and stir to coat with the oil. When the mustard seeds begin to pop, add the cabbage and snow peas. Toss the vegetables until they're well coated with the spice-infused oil. Sauté for 2 to 3 minutes, or until the cabbage begins to soften. Add the water to deglaze the pan and continue cooking until the water is absorbed. Serve immediately.

Turmeric contains curcumin, which has been shown to have similar anti-inflammatory effects as prescription medications.

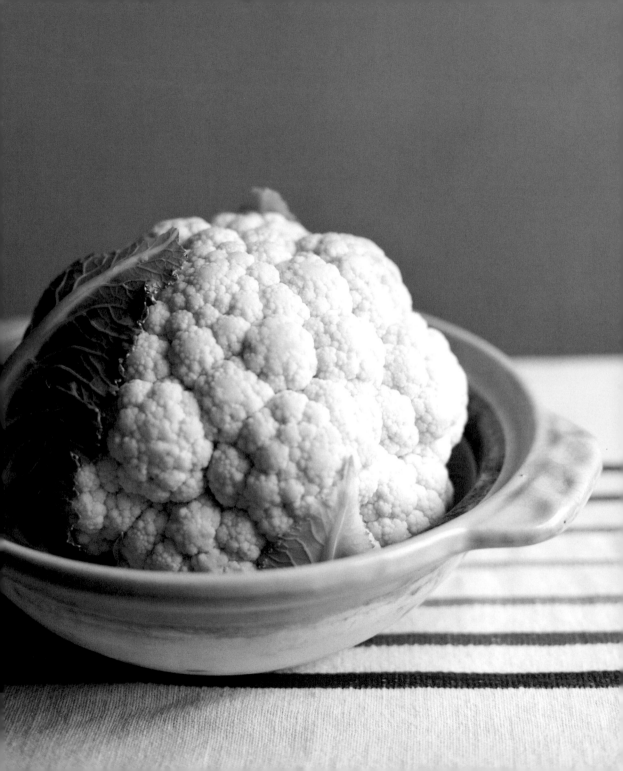

Vegetarian Main Dishes

When I'm counseling clients on anti-inflammatory eating and reviewing their food journals, there are three words that I say over, and over, *and over* again . . . eat more vegetables! In fact, I'm convinced that we would resolve the vast majority of our diet-related health issues if everyone would just take that simple advice. And I would probably be out of a job.

As an advocate for a more plant-based diet, I feel it's my responsibility to make vegetable eating not just tolerable, but downright enjoyable. I often encourage clients to experiment with just one or two meatless meals per week, so they can discover how satisfying a vegetarian or vegan dish can be. Whether you're a vegan or a meat-loving omnivore, this chapter will help you think outside the produce box. Have you ever made noodles from squash? Or used collards like a tortilla? Or created a pizza crust from cauliflower and sweet potatoes? Well hold on to your apron strings because things are about to get pretty wild in the kitchen!

Spaghetti Squash Primavera with Basil Walnut Pesto

This is the perfect recipe for the squash skeptic and is usually a hit with the kids. When you scrape out those spaghetti-like strands, it seems like something magical is happening. Using walnuts in the pesto provides a more sophisticated flavor and amps up the anti-inflammatory benefits of this dish.

Makes 4 servings

½ cup water
1 small spaghetti squash, halved
   lengthwise and seeded
¾ cup raw walnuts
2 cups packed fresh basil leaves
2 cloves garlic
½ cup plus 1 tablespoon extra-virgin
   olive oil, divided
½ teaspoon sea salt

1 cup sliced cremini mushrooms
1½ cups coarsely chopped broccoli
2 medium carrots, chopped
½ cup vegetable broth
1 cup fresh or frozen peas
½ pound fresh spinach, thoroughly
   washed
Freshly ground black pepper

Preheat the oven to 350 degrees F.

Pour the water into a shallow baking dish and place the squash in the water face down. Cover with foil and bake for 45 to 50 minutes, or until the squash is tender. Meanwhile, lightly toast the walnuts in a dry sauté pan over medium-low heat for about 5 minutes. Combine the walnuts, basil, garlic, ½ cup of the olive oil, and salt in a food processor and blend until smooth. Set aside.

In a large skillet over medium heat, add the remaining 1 tablespoon olive oil and mushrooms. Cover and cook until the mushrooms are tender, 2 to 3 minutes. Add the broccoli, carrots, and broth and sauté for 5 to 7 minutes, or until broccoli is just starting to get tender (do not overcook). Reduce the heat to low and add the peas and spinach.

Use a fork to scrape the squash flesh directly into the skillet. Add the pesto and stir well to combine all ingredients. Season to taste with pepper.

Black-Eyed Peas and Forbidden Rice with Crispy Kale

This is one of my favorite variations of the "beans, greens, and grains" dishes. Delicata is a versatile winter squash with lots of personality. Not only is it perfectly sweet, but the skin is thinner than most winter squashes, so you don't have to peel it before roasting. The combination of sweetness from the squash and savory notes from the roasted mushrooms create the perfect party when they're nestled into forbidden rice and mingling with black-eyed peas. The crunchy kale is the crowning jewel, and it's a great excuse to make up a tray of kale chips to snack on while you're waiting for dinner.

Makes 6 servings

1 head garlic
3½ tablespoons extra-virgin olive oil, divided
1 bunch curly kale, stemmed and torn into 2-inch pieces
4 teaspoons coarse sea salt, divided
1 delicata squash, ends trimmed and halved lengthwise

6 cremini mushrooms, quartered
2 tablespoons grapeseed oil
1 cup vegetable broth
½ cup forbidden rice
2 tablespoons balsamic vinegar
1 cup canned black-eyed peas, rinsed and drained

Preheat the oven to 350 degrees F.

Slice the top off the head of garlic to expose the cloves. Drizzle with ½ teaspoon of the olive oil and wrap the head in foil. Place in the oven to one side of the middle rack.

Toss the kale with a scant 1½ tablespoons olive oil, spread on a baking pan, and sprinkle with 1 teaspoon of the salt. Bake for about 12 minutes, or until the kale starts to brown and become crispy. Set aside (feel free to do some snacking!). Leave the garlic in the oven.

Increase the oven temperature to 400 degrees F.

Scoop the seeds from the squash with a spoon and cut the flesh into 1-inch chunks. Toss the squash and mushrooms with the grapeseed oil and 2 teaspoons of the salt until well coated. Spread the vegetables on a baking pan and bake for 20 minutes, or until the squash is tender and begins to caramelize. Remove the vegetables and garlic from the oven and set aside.

Meanwhile, bring the broth and rice to a boil in a medium saucepan over medium-high heat. Reduce the heat to low, cover, and simmer for 30 minutes.

Squeeze the garlic cloves into a small bowl. Stir in the remaining 2 tablespoons olive oil, balsamic vinegar, and remaining 1 teaspoon salt.

In a large bowl, combine the roasted vegetables, rice, and black-eyed peas. Drizzle with the garlic mixture and toss well to coat. Crumble the crispy kale over the top right before serving.

> Delicata squash contains anti-inflammatory phytonutrients, and it's also rich in antioxidants like beta-carotene and vitamin C.

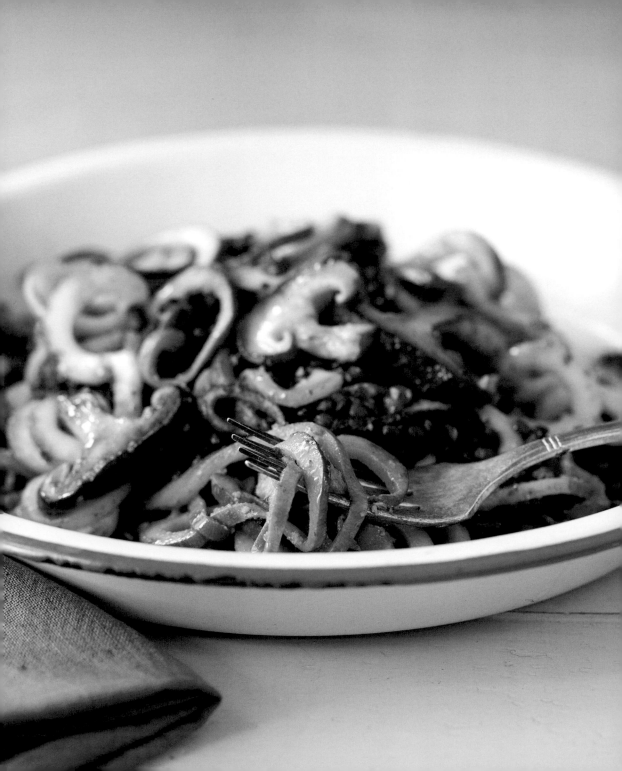

Zucchini Noodles with Pistachio Pesto and Black Lentils

It took many years of cooking for me to truly appreciate the versatility of zucchini, and I wasn't that big of a fan until I discovered zucchini noodles. It makes a pasta-inspired dish that's gluten-free, and it's just a fun way to transform an overused vegetable. This no-pasta noodle dish also features the oh-so-adorable black lentil, also known as the Beluga lentil for it's caviar-like appearance. If you cook the lentils al dente, they will retain their shape, and this will look like the most expensive faux pasta dish ever served. And you'll be dishing up one more surprise when you use pistachios in place of pine nuts in the pesto. Delicious!

Makes 6 servings

1½ cups vegetable broth, divided	1 teaspoon sea salt, divided
½ cup dried black lentils, rinsed and drained	¼ cup plus 2 teaspoons extra-virgin olive oil, divided
1 cup packed basil leaves	¼ cup water
¼ cup shelled pistachio nuts	3 medium zucchini, ends trimmed
1 small clove garlic	8 shiitake mushrooms, thinly sliced

Place 1¼ cups of the broth and lentils in a medium saucepan and bring to a boil over medium-high heat. Reduce the heat to low, cover, and simmer for 15 minutes for al dente.

Meanwhile, put the basil, pistachios, garlic, and ½ teaspoon of the salt in a food processor. With the machine running, drizzle in ¼ cup of the oil, then slowly add the water until the pesto is slightly thinner than olive oil. Set aside.

Use a spiral vegetable slicer with a 3-millimeter blade to shred the zucchini into noodles. (Alternatively, you can hand slice the zucchini or use a peeler. Cut the zucchini in half or in thirds, then slice into very thin strips.)

continued

Drizzle the remaining 2 teaspoons oil in a large skillet or sauté pan over medium heat and add the mushrooms and remaining ½ teaspoon salt. Sauté for 3 to 4 minutes, or until the mushrooms start to soften. Add the remaining ¼ cup broth and zucchini noodles to the skillet. Use tongs to gently toss the noodles with the mushrooms. Sauté for 5 minutes, or until the zucchini just begins to soften. Remove from the heat and stir in the lentils and pesto until well combined. Serve warm.

Pistachios contain high amounts of antioxidants that support the immune system, as well as specific phytonutrients called proanthocyanidins that help reduce inflammation.

Portobello Mushrooms with Samosa Filling

Not only are portobello mushrooms juicy, delicious, and nutritious, they are also the perfect vessel for a hearty samosa-style filling made from garnet yams and green peas. This can be a satisfying vegan meal, or you can use cremini mushrooms and serve it as an appetizer. It's pleasing to the eye and the palate!

Makes 2 servings

- 2 portobello mushrooms, stemmed and cleaned
- 3 tablespoons grapeseed or sunflower oil, divided
- 1 teaspoon sea salt
- 1 shallot, minced
- 1 garnet yam, peeled and chopped into 1-inch chunks
- 1 cup vegetable or mushroom broth, divided
- ¾ cup fresh or frozen peas

Preheat the oven to 350 degrees F.

With a basting brush, coat the portobellos with 2 tablespoons of the oil, seasons with the salt, and place on a baking pan. Bake for about 20 minutes, turning the mushrooms halfway through cooking.

Meanwhile, heat the remaining 1 tablespoon oil in a sauté pan over medium heat. Add the shallot and sauté for 2 to 3 minutes, or until it starts to caramelize. Add the yams and ½ cup of the broth. Cover and simmer, stirring occasionally, until the yams are soft, about 10 minutes.

Transfer the yam mixture to a food processor, add the remaining ½ cup broth, and blend until smooth. (Alternatively, you can fork-mash the mixture.) Transfer to a medium bowl.

In a small saucepan over medium heat, add the peas and enough water to cover. Bring to a gentle boil, then drain the peas and stir into the yams. Spoon the mixture into the mushroom caps and serve immediately.

Puttanesca-Style Beans and Greens

This recipe was inspired by my good friend Greg Janssen, who tried a similar dish at a local restaurant and became obsessed with trying to recreate it at home. While I never got to taste the original, I am assured that this comes very close. A secret ingredient that I added when I wanted to put my own spin on it is sun-dried tomatoes, which really elevates the flavor with an acidic sweetness. The anchovies are optional, but I really encourage adding them for the lovely saltiness they offer and also for their delightful oiliness that make them a good anti-inflammatory food. You could also top this dish with a few sardines for good measure.

Makes 6 servings

3 cups water
1 cup dried baby lima beans, soaked overnight
1 (6-inch) strip kombu (optional)
1 cup pitted kalamata olives
¾ cup pitted green olives
½ cup sun-dried tomatoes in olive oil (optional)
½ large yellow onion

2 teaspoons capers
6 tablespoons extra-virgin olive oil, divided
2 cups shredded greens (kale, chard, dandelion greens, or beet greens all work well)
4 anchovies, or 1 to 2 teaspoons anchovy paste (optional)
1 to 2 cloves garlic

In a large pot, combine the water, lima beans, and kombu and bring to a boil over high heat. Reduce the heat to medium-low, cover, and simmer for about 40 minutes, or until the beans are tender. Drain the beans and discard the kombu.

Meanwhile, in a food processor or blender, combine the olives, sun-dried tomatoes, onion, and capers and pulse until the mixture is coarsely chopped.

In a large skillet, heat 2 tablespoons of the oil over medium heat. Add the olive mixture and sauté for about 5 minutes, or until the onions start to become translucent. Add the greens, anchovies, and garlic and sauté for 3 to 4 minutes. Stir in the beans until well incorporated. Serve warm or at room temperature.

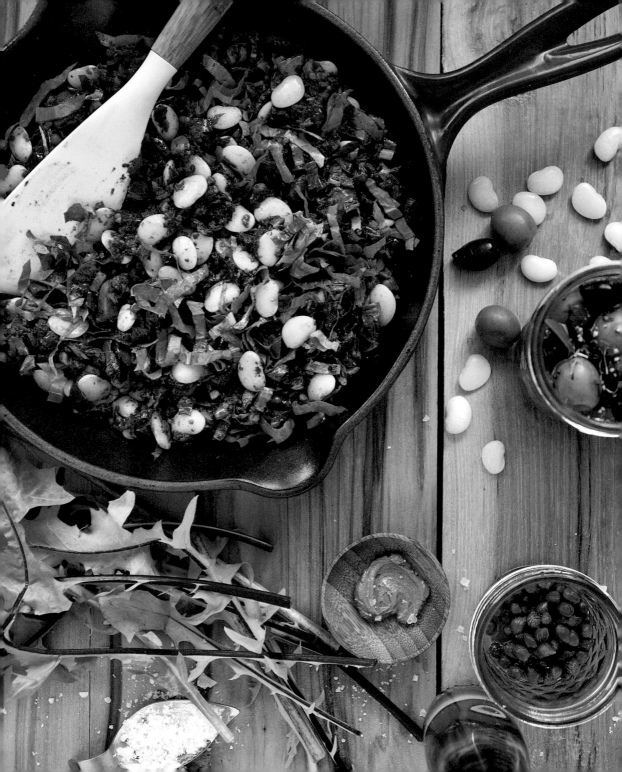

Toasted Pecan Quinoa Burgers

Toasted pecans have a sweet, earthy flavor that helps to make these meat-free "burgers" unique. The quinoa lends itself to the nutty flavor of the pecans and rounds out the nutritional profile of these tasty burgers. When I want to have a more "burger-like" experience, I put this on a gluten-free bun with lettuce, tomatoes, and onion, or sometimes I just place the patty between two large lettuce leaves. Serve these to your vegan friends and watch them savor every bite!

Makes 8 servings

¾ cup pecans
2¼ cups vegetable broth, divided
1 cup quinoa, rinsed and drained
1 teaspoon sea salt, plus more for
    seasoning
½ cup sunflower seeds
¼ cup sesame seeds
1 teaspoon ground cumin

1 teaspoon dried oregano
1 carrot, shredded
½ cup canned black beans, rinsed and
    drained
Freshly ground black pepper
1 teaspoon coconut or sunflower oil
1 avocado, thinly sliced

Preheat the oven to 375 degrees F.

Spread the pecans on a baking pan and roast for 5 to 7 minutes.

Combine 2 cups of the broth, quinoa, and salt in a large saucepan and bring to a boil over medium-high heat. Reduce the heat to low, cover, and simmer for 20 minutes without stirring. Measure 1 cup of the quinoa for use in the burgers, reserving any extra for another use.

Combine the pecans, sunflower seeds, sesame seeds, cumin, and oregano in a food processor and grind to a medium-coarse texture.

In a large bowl, stir together the 1 cup quinoa, nut mixture, carrot, and beans. While stirring, slowly add the remaining ¼ cup broth until mixture becomes tacky. Season to taste with salt and pepper.

Form the mixture into 8 patties about ½-inch thick and cook, refrigerate, or freeze immediately.

Heat the coconut oil in a large skillet over medium-high heat. Add half of the patties and cook for about 2 minutes on each side (cook longer from frozen). Repeat with the remaining patties. Top the burgers with avocado slices.

Quinoa is the only grain that is considered a complete protein, and it also contains a small amount of omega-3s.

Hearty Mushroom and Lentil Stew

The combination of mushrooms and lentils makes for a hearty, satisfying stew that even meat lovers enjoy. I like to make a big batch when I have company for the weekend, so we can heat it up for a quick lunch or serve it over quinoa with some sautéed greens for dinner. Any type of black, brown, or green lentil will work in this stew, and you can also play around with different types of mushrooms. I've used chanterelles and porcinis and had good results.

Makes 8 servings

2 teaspoons sunflower oil
2 cups diced red onion
1 cup chopped celery
1 cup chopped carrots
2 cloves garlic, minced
1 bay leaf
5 cups sliced shiitake mushrooms
1½ cups sliced portobello mushrooms

½ cup dried French lentils
1 quart mushroom broth
2 tablespoons cooking sherry
Sea salt and freshly ground black pepper
¼ cup chopped fresh parsley, for garnish

Heat the oil in large soup pot or Dutch oven over medium heat. Add the onion and sauté for 5 minutes, or until tender. Add the celery, carrots, garlic, and bay leaf and sauté, stirring frequently, for 10 minutes, or until the onion is golden brown. Stir in the mushrooms and sauté for 10 minutes, or until most of the liquid has evaporated. Stir in the lentils, broth, and sherry. Season to taste with salt and pepper. Bring the mixture to a boil, then reduce the heat to medium-low, cover, and simmer for 30 to 40 minutes, or until the lentils are tender.

Discard the bay leaf. Ladle the stew into individual bowls, sprinkle with the parsley, and serve.

Southwestern-Style Buckwheat Polenta Stacks

Buckwheat fascinates me. Even though it has "wheat" in its name, it's actually not a grain at all. It's related to rhubarb and is safe for those who are avoiding gluten. It also happens to be a good source of tryptophan, so you might just find that you sleep like a baby after this nutritious meal! Buckwheat has a characteristically strong flavor, but I think it works nicely with the spicy bean mixture in this recipe. It also makes a great alternative to corn polenta, which takes much longer to cook and requires a lot of stirring. You can get creative with the bean mixture: I love to add roasted red peppers.

Makes 9 buckwheat stacks

2 cups water
1 cup toasted buckwheat groats
¼ teaspoon sea salt
2 teaspoons extra-virgin olive oil
1 small onion, diced
1 (15-ounce) can pinto beans with
   liquid
2 teaspoons maple syrup

1 teaspoon ground cumin
1 teaspoon garlic powder
1 teaspoon dried oregano
½ teaspoon paprika
¼ teaspoon cayenne pepper
2 cups chopped spinach
1 avocado, thinly sliced

In a large saucepan, bring the water to a boil. Add the groats and salt, reduce the heat to low, cover, and simmer for 10 minutes.

Transfer the groats to a food processor and blend. Texture will be somewhat rough and thick, like polenta. Allow the mixture to cool slightly for a couple minutes.

Take a small handful of the buckwheat mixture—the size of a large meatball—roll it, and then flatten onto a baking pan. Press each disk to a ¼-inch thickness. Repeat until you have used all of the buckwheat mixture.

continued

Drizzle the oil in a large skillet, add the onion, and stir until well coated. Place the skillet over medium heat and sauté the onion until translucent. Add the beans, maple syrup, cumin, garlic powder, oregano, paprika, and cayenne. Stir well and sauté for 3 to 5 minutes. Use potato masher or fork to smash some of the beans, allowing some to remain whole. The mixture should be the consistency of chunky refried beans.

Place a small handful of spinach on a buckwheat cake. Scoop a generous amount of the bean mixture over the spinach. Top with avocado slices. Repeat with the rest of the buckwheat cakes.

Tip: For a crispy cake, before stacking, place the buckwheat rounds under the broiler for 3 minutes on each side.

Quinoa-Stuffed Collard Rolls

Collard greens are most commonly used in southern dishes. They're generally cooked with bacon, ham, or some form of pork that lends saltiness and cuts the bitterness that's inherent to this member of the cabbage family. The savory quinoa filling and rich, buttery flavor of the toasted pecans also helps disguise the bitterness of the greens—no pork required. You can save some time if you have large, pliable collard leaves that are flexible enough to roll without blanching. You can also choose to skip the step of baking the finished rolls if you want the benefit of eating the greens raw. Steaming in the oven just helps soften the collards a bit more and may make them more desirable for those who are still on the fence about these mysterious greens.

Makes 6 servings

2½ cups vegetable broth, divided	¾ cup chopped mushrooms
1 cup quinoa	2 carrots, shredded
1 bunch collard greens, washed with stems removed	1 clove garlic
	1 teaspoon ground sage
½ cup pecans	1 teaspoon dried oregano
1 tablespoon grapeseed oil	2 teaspoons sea salt
1 small onion, diced	

In a medium saucepan, add 2 cups of the broth and quinoa and bring to a boil over medium-high heat. Reduce the heat to low, cover, and simmer for 20 minutes without stirring. Fluff with a fork and let cool for about 5 minutes.

Preheat the oven to 350 degrees F.

Bring a large pot of water to a boil. Add the collard greens and blanch for 2 minutes. Drain and rinse with cold water. Set aside.

Place the pecans in a small dry sauté pan and toast over medium heat until they become aromatic and start to brown slightly. Coarsely chop the nuts.

continued

Heat the oil in a large sauté pan over medium heat. Add the onion and sauté until translucent. Add the mushrooms and sauté for 2 minutes. Add the carrots, garlic, sage, and oregano and sauté for 3 minutes. Stir in the quinoa, pecans, and salt.

Place a generous scoop of filling onto a collard leaf. Roll the leaf burrito-style and place seam down in a square baking dish. Repeat until all the collards and filling have been used. Pour the remaining ½ cup broth over the rolls, cover with foil, and bake for 25 minutes.

Collard greens are right up there with kale when it comes to outstanding anti-inflammatory foods. They're an excellent source of vitamin K, which directly regulates the body's inflammatory response, as well as a good source of omega-3s.

Golden Beet and Mushroom Faux Gratin

I don't like to play favorites, but this recipe is certainly a contender for first place in my book. It really is the whole package: the sweet earthiness of the roasted beets, the savory succulence of the portobellos, and the tangy, nutty creaminess of the layers in between. The gratin is extremely rich and surprisingly filling, but it's still hard for me to put down my fork. I'm hoping this dish will result in a slew of beet-loving converts!

Makes 6 servings

1 cup raw cashews
½ cup unsweetened almond milk
2 tablespoons tahini
2 tablespoons nutritional yeast
1 tablespoon freshly squeezed
    lemon juice
1½ teaspoons coarse sea salt, divided

1 teaspoon garlic powder
4 medium unpeeled golden beets,
    well scrubbed and ends trimmed
2 large portobello mushrooms
2 tablespoons extra-virgin olive oil,
    divided

Preheat the oven to 425 degrees F.

In a food processor, finely chop the cashews. Add the almond milk, tahini, nutritional yeast, lemon juice, ½ teaspoon of the salt, and garlic powder. Blend until the mixture is the consistency of creamy peanut butter, adding water as needed. Set aside.

Slice the beets into ¼-inch-thick slices (a mandolin works well for this). Cut the portobellos into large ¼-inch-thick slices.

Drizzle 1 tablespoon of the oil in a 9-by-12-inch baking dish. Arrange one layer of beets along the bottom of the dish. Arrange a layer of mushrooms over the beets. Spread half of the cashew mixture over the mushrooms. Arrange another layer of beets on top of the nut spread and repeat the layering ingredients in this order (it's best to end with a layer of mushrooms). Drizzle the remaining 1 tablespoon oil over the top layer and sprinkle with the remaining 1 teaspoon salt. Cover and bake for 55 minutes. Serve warm.

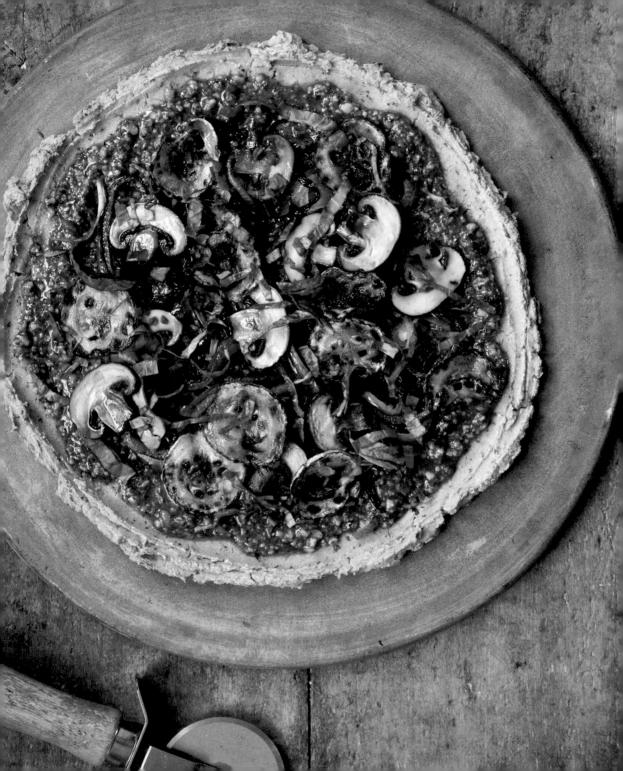

Veggie Pizza with Cauliflower-Yam Crust

If I were to take a poll and ask my gluten-free, dairy-free clients what food they miss the most, I'm certain that pizza would easily top the list. I've played around with dozens of variations of a gluten-free crust and topped them with some pretty pathetic cheese wannabes, but nothing comes close to the real thing. What I love about this veggie pizza is that it's not trying to be a big, doughy, cheesy pizza when it grows up. It's entirely unique, with a vegetable-based crust, pesto in place of cheese, and succulent sautéed vegetables on top. It's quite tasty the next day, and who wouldn't want to eat cold pizza for breakfast and have it be healthy!

Makes 4 servings

½ medium head cauliflower, broken into small florets
½ medium garnet yam, peeled and chopped into ½-inch chunks
1 tablespoon dried Italian herbs
¾ teaspoon sea salt, divided
1 cup brown rice flour

1 tablespoon coconut oil, plus more for greasing pizza stone
1 small red onion, sliced into thin rings
½ cup sliced cremini mushrooms
1 yellow summer squash or zucchini
2 cups spinach
¼ to ½ cup vegan pesto (store-bought is OK)

Preheat the oven to 400 degrees F. If you have a pizza stone, put it in the oven.

Place a steamer basket in a large pot with 1 inch of water. Put the cauliflower and yam in the basket and steam until both are easily pierced with a fork, about 15 minutes. Do not overcook or the vegetables will be too wet.

Transfer the vegetables to a food processor. Add the Italian herbs and ½ teaspoon of the salt and blend until smooth. Transfer the mixture to a large bowl. Gradually add the flour, stirring until the mixture is well combined.

continued

Grease the pizza stone or a pizza pan with coconut oil. Pile the cauliflower mixture in the center of the pizza stone. Use a spatula to carefully spread the "dough" evenly in a circular pattern (much like spreading frosting) until the crust is about ⅛ inch thick. Bake for 40 to 45 minutes. Turn on the broiler and broil the crust for 2 minutes to make the top crispy (watch carefully to avoid burning).

Meanwhile, heat the coconut oil in a medium skillet over medium heat. Add the onion and sauté for 2 minutes. Add the mushrooms, squash, and remaining ¼ teaspoon salt and sauté for 3 to 4 minutes. Stir in the spinach and remove from the heat just as it begins to wilt.

Spread the pesto evenly over the pizza crust. Spread the sautéed vegetables over the pesto. Slice the pizza, it's ready to serve!

Tip: The cauliflower crust serves as a great stand-in for flatbread and can even be used to make sandwiches.

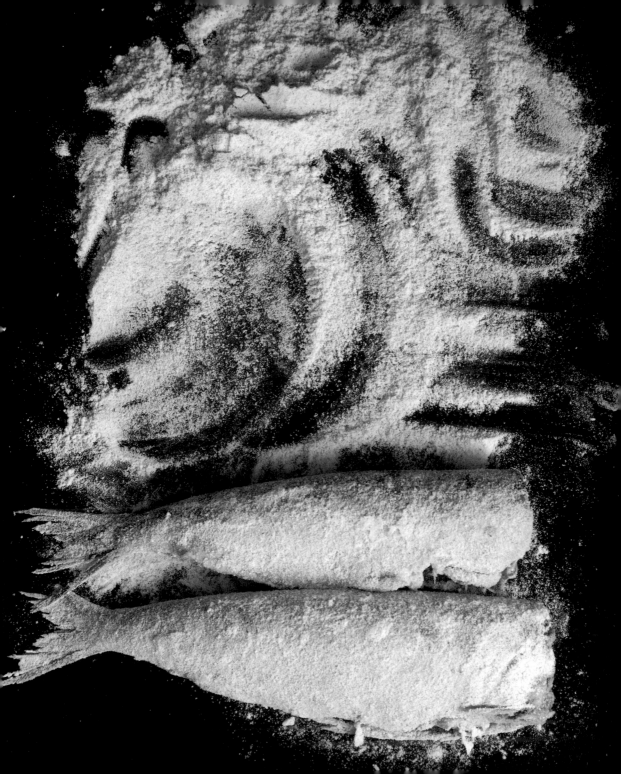

Pescatarian Main Dishes

One of the hallmarks of a Mediterranean diet is that the primary source of animal protein is fish. As we start to gain a better understanding of the role inflammation plays in the development of various diseases, it becomes more obvious why populations eating more fish and vegetables tend to be healthier. We know that oily finfish, like salmon, halibut, mackerel, and sardines, are rich sources of inflammation-blocking omega-3s.

When I give clients the recommendation to eat fish three to four times per week, they often tell me that they're just not confident about cooking it. So it should come as a relief that fish is actually one of the easiest, quick-cooking forms of protein out there. It takes less time to prepare than chicken. It's more versatile than beef. And there are a variety of cooking methods that can guarantee perfect results every time. It just takes some practice. The recipes in this chapter will encourage you to try poaching, roasting, pan-frying, and steaming in parchment. Be fearless in your attempts, and any insecurities about being able to cook fish correctly will soon be overcome.

Another concern that's often raised about seafood is sustainability and accumulation of heavy metals (like mercury) and other contaminants. That's why it's important to choose your fish wisely. One of the best resources I've found is the Monterey Bay Aquarium's Seafood Watch Program. You can visit their website or download the app and see which types of fish are the best bets.

Hazelnut-Encrusted Halibut with Dipping Sauce

I like to think of this as a healthier, anti-inflammatory version of fish and chips. Hazelnuts have a buttery sweetness when roasted, and they make a delicious bread-free crust. You won't get the golden-brown coloration and crispy texture of battered and fried fish, but you'll still get good flavor and a lot more anti-inflammatory unsaturated fats. The dipping sauce is reminiscent of tartar sauce. Just throw in some oven-roasted sweet potatoes fries and the package will be complete!

Makes 4 servings

1 cup raw hazelnuts
¼ cup brown rice flour
1 tablespoon Italian herbs
½ teaspoon sea salt
1½ pounds halibut or any other firm white fish, skin removed and cut into 4 fillets
3 tablespoons extra-virgin olive oil

FOR THE SAUCE:
½ cup Soy-Free Vegenaise
½ teaspoon Dijon or stone-ground mustard
1 small dill pickle, finely chopped
1 teaspoon pickle juice
½ teaspoon honey
¼ teaspoon freshly grated lemon zest

Preheat the oven to 350 degrees F.

Spread the hazelnuts on a baking sheet and roast for 10 minutes. Transfer the nuts to a clean dish towel while they're still warm. Wrap the pile of nuts in the towel and aggressively massage them to remove the bitter skins. When the nuts are cool to the touch, transfer to a food processor and pulse until finely chopped. (Alternatively, put the hazelnuts in a plastic bag, seal, and use a meat tenderizer to pound them into fine crumbs.

Combine the hazelnuts, flour, Italian herbs, and salt in a shallow dish. Use a basting brush to coat both sides of the halibut fillets with the oil and then carefully press each fillet in the hazelnut mixture, making sure both sides are thoroughly coated.

continued

Place the halibut in a baking dish and bake for 15 to 20 minutes. The fish should be just opaque but not dry.

Meanwhile to make the sauce, whisk together the Vegenaise, mustard, pickle, pickle juice, honey, and lemon zest.

Place a small spoonful of sauce on each fillet or serve on the side for dipping.

Halibut and other types of oily white fish are great sources of omega-3s and magnesium, a winning combination for reducing inflammation and protecting the heart.

Poached White Fish with Mango Lime Chutney

Poaching fish is perhaps the easiest of all cooking methods. It also guarantees that the fish will stay moist because you're immersing it in liquid. And it saves you the trouble of removing the skin from the fish because it will just slide right off after cooking. The mango lime chutney helps brighten up the dish and makes you feel like you're dining on the beach in the tropics (or at least you can pretend).

Makes 4 servings

FOR THE CHUTNEY:
1 mango, peeled, pitted, and diced
1 small shallot, minced
1 teaspoon minced peeled ginger
¼ cup finely chopped fresh cilantro
2 tablespoons freshly squeezed lime juice
½ teaspoon sea salt

1 cup vegetable broth
1 cup water
1½ pounds white fish (halibut, cod, or black cod), cut into 4 fillets
1 teaspoon sea salt
½ teaspoon freshly ground black pepper

To make the chutney, in medium bowl, stir together the mango, shallot, ginger, cilantro, lime juice, and salt. Set aside to allow the flavors to mingle.

In a deep cast-iron skillet or saucepan, bring the broth and water to a gentle boil over medium-high heat. Place fillets in the skillet and season with the salt and pepper. Cover and reduce the heat to medium. Poach for 8 to 9 minutes. The fish should be opaque in the center but still moist.

Carefully transfer the fillets from the skillet to plates, leaving the skin behind. Top with the chutney and serve.

Tip: Prepare an extra fillet and reserve some chutney for a fish taco the next day. I like to serve mine with Brussels Sprout Slaw (page 98).

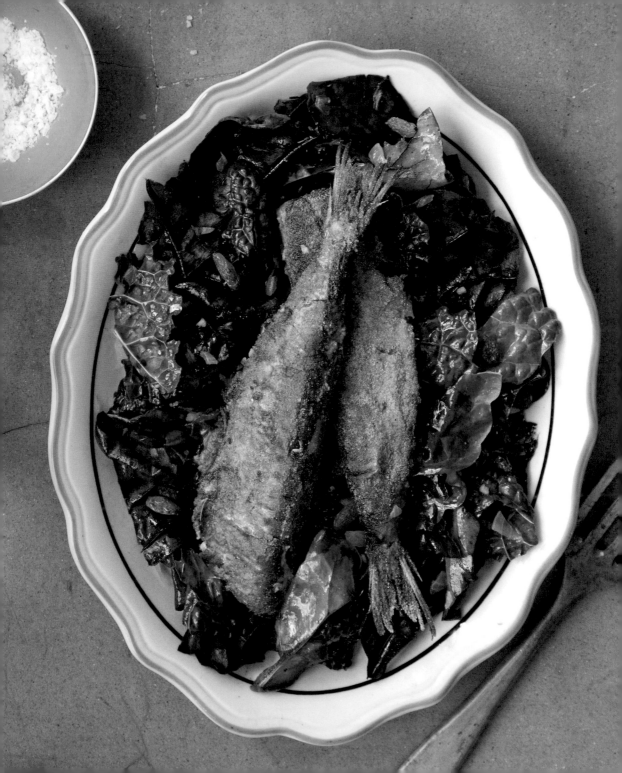

Pan-Fried Sardines with Sautéed Kale and Chard

Sardines. You either love 'em or you hate 'em. I've been on a crusade to try to convert the masses, but I have to admit, it's slowgoing. For me, sardines have always been an easy sell. I used to sit on my grandpa's lap and we'd eat canned sardines with a row of Ritz crackers. As an adult (and a nutritionist), I've come to appreciate the fabulous anti-inflammatory qualities of sardines. They're one of the most concentrated sources of omega-3 fatty acids, and they're also low on the food chain, so they don't accumulate mercury or other contaminants. This meal, featuring sardines and kale, would rank at the top of all the anti-inflammatory dishes in this book. Have I converted you yet?

Makes 4 servings

¾ cup brown rice flour
2 teaspoons curry powder
1 teaspoon ground cumin
1 pound fresh sardines, cleaned, scaled, and heads removed
1 tablespoon grapeseed or sunflower oil

1 small yellow onion, diced
1 bunch kale, stemmed and chopped
1 bunch chard, stemmed and chopped
1 clove garlic, chopped
¼ cup vegetable broth
¼ cup golden raisins

In a shallow baking dish, whisk together the flour, curry powder, and cumin. Dredge the sardines in the flour mixture until well coated.

Heat the oil in a cast-iron skillet over medium-high heat. When hot, add the sardines to the skillet in batches and cook for 1½ to 2 minutes per side. Transfer the sardines to a plate lined with paper towels. Repeat with the remaining sardines, adding more oil to the skillet as needed.

Reduce the heat to medium and add the onion to the skillet. Sauté for 4 to 5 minutes, or until the onion starts to sweat and soften. Add kale, chard, and garlic. Deglaze the pan with the broth and cook the greens until they begin to wilt, 2 to 3 minutes. Stir in the raisins. Divide the greens among each plate and top with the sardines.

Salmon en Papillote with Silky Celery Root Puree

Cooking fish in parchment is a foolproof way to ensure perfectly cooked fish that's moist. The celery root puree is smooth and silky, resembling expertly blended mashed potatoes but with a completely different flavor profile. Adding sunchokes (also called Jerusalem artichokes) to the puree gives it a bit of a nutty essence. If you can't find sunchokes, try parsnips instead. The salmon fillets look beautiful resting on pillows of pureed goodness. All you need to do is add some greens to create the ideal anti-inflammatory plate!

Makes 4 servings

1½ pounds salmon, bones removed and cut into 4 fillets
1 lemon, halved
1 teaspoon sea salt
1 teaspoon celery seed
¼ cup chopped Italian parsley or celery leaves, for garnish (optional)

FOR THE PUREE:
1 medium celeriac (celery root), peeled and cut into 1-inch chunks
4 sunchokes, thoroughly scrubbed and cut into 1-inch chunks
1½ cups vegetable broth
1 teaspoon sea salt
Freshly ground black pepper

Preheat the oven to 350 degrees F.

Cut sheets of parchment paper into 4 large heart-shaped pieces that can cover each fillet. Place a fillet on each parchment heart, slightly off center. Season each fillet with a squeeze of lemon juice, ¼ teaspoon salt, and ¼ teaspoon celery seed. Fold the parchment over the fillet so all edges of the paper meet. Working your way around parchment, fold the edges over twice and end with a twist at the bottom of the heart. The fillets should be well sealed inside the paper so no steam escapes.

Place the packages on a baking pan and bake for 15 to 20 minutes.

Meanwhile, to make the puree, place a steamer basket in a pot with 1 inch of water. Put the celeriac and sunchokes in the basket and steam until tender, about 15 minutes. Transfer the vegetables to a food processor, add the broth and salt, and blend until smooth. Season to taste with pepper.

Carefully remove the fish from the parchment paper. Put a generous scoop of the puree on a plate. Place a fillet on top of the puree. Garnish with the parsley and serve with a side of sautéed greens.

In addition to being a great source of omega-3s, salmon contains unique bioactive proteins that may be particularly effective in reducing joint inflammation.

Mediterranean Salmon Skewers

There's something about putting food on skewers that almost immediately makes it more interesting to eat. I love using salmon when making these skewers in the spring and summer months, and I'm more inclined to use lamb in fall and winter. You can choose which type of protein you'd like to use (the marinade works well on most types of fish, meat, or poultry) and then switch up the veggies for a whole new experience. I find that it helps to put your picky eaters to work on the skewer assembly line so they can custom-make a couple skewers with their favorite ingredients.

Makes 8 servings

½ cup extra-virgin olive oil
1 tablespoon freshly squeezed lime
  juice
1 teaspoon freshly grated lime zest
1 clove garlic, minced
2 tablespoons chopped fresh oregano
1 tablespoon chopped fresh mint
1 teaspoon sea salt
¾ pound salmon, skin and bones
  removed, cut into 1½-inch cubes

12 cremini mushrooms, quartered
1 small head broccoli, broken
  into florets
1 summer squash or zucchini, cut into
  1-inch chunks
½ cup pitted kalamata olives
8 wooden skewers, soaked in water
  for at least 30 minutes

Preheat the oven to 375 degrees F.

In a medium bowl, combine the oil, lime juice and zest, garlic, oregano, mint, and salt.

Combine the salmon, mushrooms, broccoli, and squash in a baking dish. Drizzle with the marinade and gently toss until the salmon and vegetables are well coated.

Layer the salmon, vegetables, and olives on the skewers, alternating the order on each skewer.

Place the skewers on a broiler pan and bake for 20 to 25 minutes, turning them halfway through cooking.

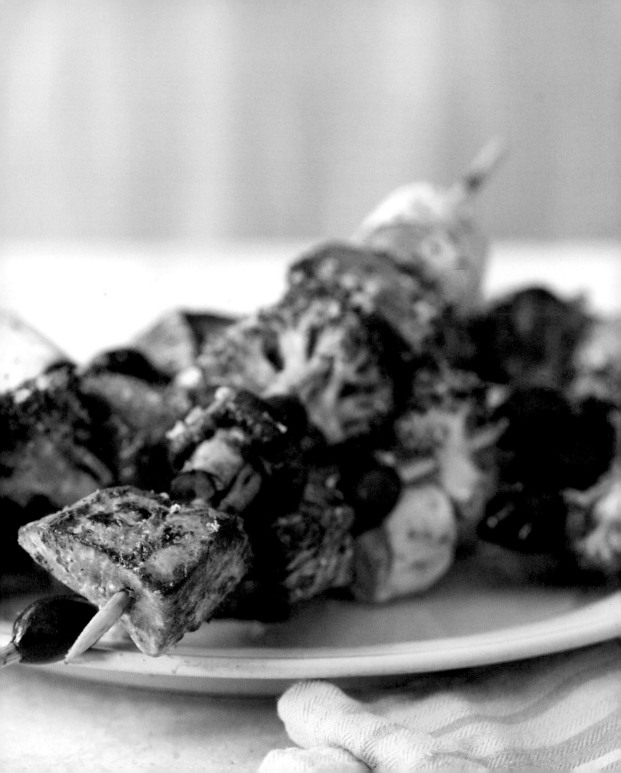

Pumpkin Coconut Curry with White Fish

Just saying "pumpkin coconut curry" out loud makes my mouth water in anticipation. I created this recipe for a cooking class I was teaching in the fall, and it quickly became a favorite among the class participants and the cooking assistants. If you like pumpkin and you are a fan of curry, you'll love this dish. The rich, complex flavors of the pumpkin and coconut unite with the earthy heat of the curry and cayenne to create the perfect balance of flavors. If you're still working on becoming a fish lover, this is an exquisite way to enjoy a mild white fish that will blend right in without any hopes of overpowering the sauce. I've also recreated this dish as a vegetarian meal by replacing the fish with chickpeas and adding more veggies (like mushrooms, broccoli, and cauliflower).

Makes 6 servings

2 tablespoons coconut oil
1 small yellow onion, diced
2 cloves garlic, minced
1 teaspoon minced peeled ginger
1 (15-ounce) can pumpkin puree
1 cup vegetable broth
1 cup coconut milk
1½ cups frozen peas

5 Kaffir lime leaves
2 teaspoons curry powder
¼ teaspoon cayenne pepper
1 pound white fish (halibut, cod, or black cod), skin and bones removed, cut into 1-inch cubes
2 teaspoons sea salt
Forbidden black rice, for serving

Heat the oil in a deep cast-iron skillet or saucepan over medium heat. Add the onion and sauté until translucent, about 5 minutes. Add garlic and ginger and sauté for 2 to 3 minutes. Stir in the pumpkin puree, broth, coconut milk, peas, lime leaves, curry powder, and cayenne. Reduce the heat to medium-low, add the fish and salt to the skillet, cover, and simmer for 10 to 15 minutes.

Serve the curry over forbidden black rice for a beautiful contrast of color.

Pumpkin is rich in antioxidants like beta-carotene and vitamin C, so it helps keep the immune system tuned up and prevents oxidative damage that leads to inflammation.

Sizzling Salmon and Quinoa Skillet

One-pot meals are the norm at my house. I've always enjoyed comingling the food on my plate, so why not just throw all of my favorite ingredients into a sizzling skillet and call it dinner? This dish looks like a work of art too, with its earthy tones from the mushrooms and quinoa, various shades of green, and of course the beautiful pink salmon. I make this often for impromptu dinner parties when I'm in the mood for a more rustic, casual theme, but I also love to serve it as a brunch entrée. In fact, I encourage you to eat any leftovers for breakfast. I can't think of a more balanced meal to help you kick off the day.

Makes 4 servings

1 head garlic
½ teaspoon extra-virgin olive oil
2½ cups mushroom broth, divided
1 cup quinoa, rinsed and drained
1 tablespoon coconut oil
½ pound chanterelle mushrooms, sliced
1 cup shredded brussels sprouts

1 cup frozen petite peas
2 tablespoons nutritional yeast
2 tablespoons chopped fresh basil
1 tablespoon dried oregano
½ pound salmon, skin and bones removed, cut into 1-inch cubes
Sea salt and freshly ground black pepper

Preheat the oven to 350 degrees F.

Slice the top off the head of garlic to expose the cloves. Drizzle with the olive oil and wrap the head in foil. Place in the oven and roast for 50 minutes.

Meanwhile, combine 2 cups of the broth and quinoa in large saucepan. Bring to boil over high heat, then reduce the heat to low, cover, and cook for 20 minutes without stirring. Measure 1 cup of the quinoa to use in this recipe, reserving any extra for another use.

continued

In a large skillet, heat the coconut oil over medium heat. Add the mushrooms and sauté for 5 minutes, or until they release liquid and become soft. Add the brussels sprouts and sauté for 3 minutes, adding up to ¼ cup broth as needed to prevent the mushrooms and sprouts from sticking to the skillet. Add the peas, nutritional yeast, basil, and oregano and sauté, stirring occasionally, for 5 minutes. Add the salmon to the skillet and toss gently to combine. Gently squeeze the garlic cloves into the skillet. Cover and cook, stirring occasionally, for 4 to 5 minutes.

Add the 1 cup quinoa and remaining ¼ cup broth to the skillet and stir until well combined. Season to taste with salt and pepper and serve.

Tip: A perfectly poached egg can be the crowning jewel on this skillet mix if you're heating it up for breakfast the next day.

Nori-Wrapped Mackerel with Wasabi "Mayo"

Mackerel is one of the top picks for anti-inflammatory eating. It's an oilier fish, which means it's ultra high in omega-3s. When I ask my cooking class if they ever eat mackerel, the typical response is "only in sushi." So I was inspired to create a cooked version that would be easy for the home cook. I bake fish in nori for the same reason I use parchment—it steams the fish and prevents it from drying out.

Makes 4 servings

2 cups water
1 cup brown basmati rice, rinsed and drained
¾ teaspoon sea salt, divided
2 tablespoons toasted sesame oil
1 tablespoon rice wine vinegar

½ teaspoon minced peeled ginger
1 pound mackerel, skin and bones removed
1 (1-ounce) package nori sheets
¼ cup Soy-Free Vegenaise
2 teaspoons wasabi powder

Preheat the oven to 350 degrees F.

Put the water, rice, and ¼ teaspoon of the salt in a large saucepan and bring to a boil over medium-high heat. Reduce the heat to low, cover, and simmer for 45 to 50 minutes, or until all of the water is absorbed.

Meanwhile, in a small bowl, combine the oil, vinegar, ginger, and remaining ½ teaspoon salt.

Slice the mackerel into strips about 1 inch wide by 3 inches long. Place a strip of mackerel on a sheet nori. Top with about 3 tablespoons of the rice. Drizzle the oil mixture over the rice and carefully roll the nori sheet like a burrito, folding in the ends as you go. Place the rolls in a baking dish, cover with foil, and bake for 15 minutes.

Meanwhile, in a small bowl, blend the Vegenaise and wasabi powder.

Serve the wrapped mackerel with a generous spoonful of the wasabi mayo for dipping.

Tip: Spritzing the nori sheets with a little bit of water minutes before filling makes them much more pliable and easier to roll without tearing.

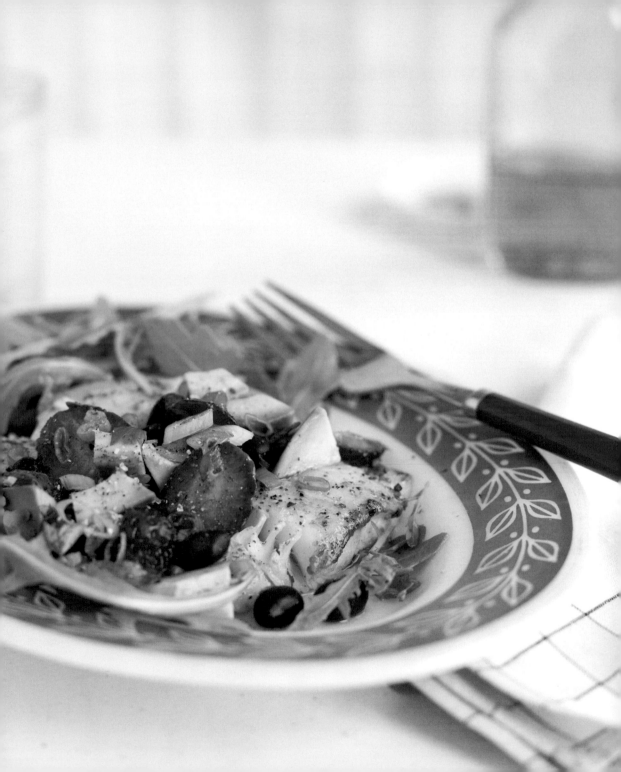

Fish Taco Salad with Strawberry Avocado Salsa

The first time I made this salsa, I had an audience of dinner guests looking on as I tossed the strawberries into a bowl with the rest of the salsa ingredients. "That's interesting" was one of the comments. "I never would have thought to put strawberries in salsa" was another. I sensed some skepticism. After a few tentative bites of the fish salad with the salsa, they were all scooping generous amounts onto their plates. The fruity salsa works well with the peppery arugula and creates a fish taco salad that surprises the skeptics. Don't forget the margaritas!

Makes 4 servings

FOR THE SALSA:
½ avocado, diced
3 strawberries, hulled and diced
¼ cup canned black beans, rinsed and drained
1 small shallot, diced
2 green onions, thinly sliced
¼ cup finely chopped fresh cilantro
1 teaspoon finely chopped peeled ginger
3 tablespoons freshly squeezed lime juice
½ teaspoon sea salt
⅛ teaspoon cayenne pepper

2 tablespoons extra-virgin olive oil or avocado oil
2 teaspoons agave nectar
1 tablespoon freshly squeezed lime juice
4 cups arugula
1½ pounds light fish (halibut, cod, or red snapper), cut into 4 fillets
1 teaspoon sea salt
½ teaspoon freshly ground black pepper

Preheat a gas or charcoal grill.

To make the salsa, in a medium bowl, combine the avocado, strawberries, beans, shallot, green onions, cilantro, ginger, lime juice, salt, and cayenne. Mix until the ingredients are well blended and set aside.

continued

To make the salad, in a small bowl, whisk together the oil, agave, and lime juice. Put the arugula in a large bowl and toss with the vinaigrette.

Season the fish fillets with the salt and pepper. Grill over direct high heat for 7 to 9 minutes, turning the fish once during cooking. The fish should be opaque and flake easily.

To serve, pile 1 cup of the arugula salad on each plate. Place a fillet on the salad and top with a heaping spoonful of salsa.

The unique combination of healthy fats and phytosterols in avocados are what make them particularly useful in reducing inflammation related to arthritis.

Oven-Roasted Black Cod with Smashed Sweet Peas

My first introduction to black cod was a rather unsuccessful grilling experience, but I'm so glad that I tried it again. Black cod, also called sablefish, is loaded with omega-3s, and it ranks high on the sustainability list. I prefer to roast or poach it, and I'm in love with the subtle, buttery flavor. Even those who are finicky about fish generally appreciate black cod. The smashed peas are such a simple side dish and they add so much to the plate. And the best part? This gourmet-looking dinner only takes twenty minutes to make.

Makes 4 servings

2 leeks (white and light green parts only), sliced into thick rings
1 pound shiitake mushrooms, sliced
2 tablespoons grapeseed oil
2 teaspoons coarse sea salt, divided, plus more for seasoning
2 pounds black cod, skin and bones removed, cut into 4 fillets

1 teaspoon freshly ground black pepper
1 teaspoon sweet paprika
1 tablespoon extra-virgin olive oil, divided
2 shallots, chopped
2 cloves garlic, chopped
2 cups fresh or frozen sweet peas
¾ cup vegetable broth

Preheat the oven to 400 degrees F.

Combine the leeks, mushrooms, grapeseed oil, and 1 teaspoon of the salt in a large bowl and toss until well coated. Spread the vegetables in a 9-by-14-inch baking dish and roast for 10 minutes.

Remove the dish from the oven and place the fish fillets on top of the vegetables. Season with the remaining 1 teaspoon salt, pepper, and paprika. Bake for 8 to 10 minutes, or until the fish flakes easily and is opaque in the center.

continued

Meanwhile, heat 2 teaspoons of the olive oil in a medium skillet over medium heat. Add the shallots and sauté for 2 to 3 minutes. Add the garlic and sauté for 2 minutes. Stir in the peas, add the remaining 1 teaspoon olive oil, and sauté for about 5 minutes.

Transfer half of the pea mixture to a blender or food processor. Drizzle in the broth and pulse until the peas begin to resemble a thick soup. Return the blended peas to the skillet, season with the salt and pepper, and stir well.

To serve, put a generous scoop of pea mash to one side of each plate; place a fish fillet in the center of the plate, slightly overlapping the smashed peas; and top with the roasted vegetables.

Not only do shiitake mushrooms contain more than a hundred compounds that may help prevent cancer, they also keep our blood vessels healthy and block inflammation that can lead to heart disease.

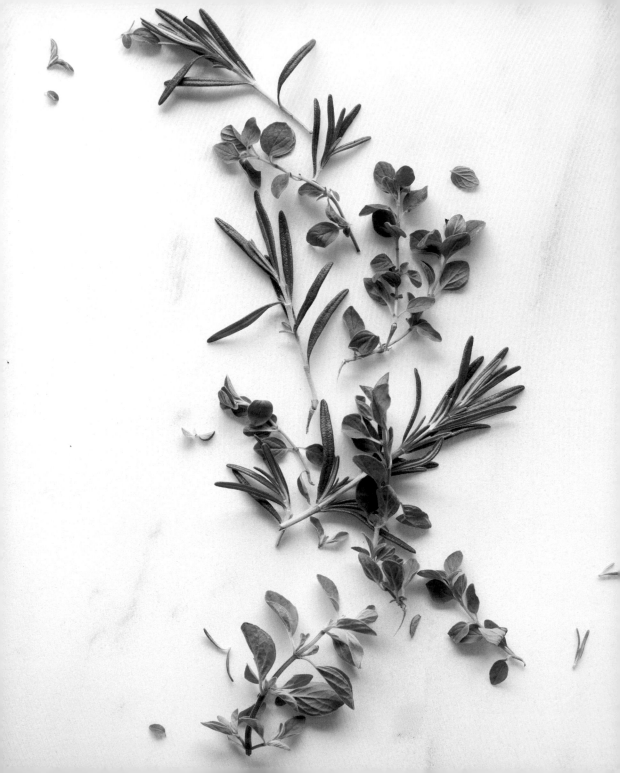

Hint-of-Meat
Main Dishes

While eating copious amounts of meat and poultry can lead to more inflammation, there's definitely a way to include them as part of the Mediterranean-style diet. It's called moderation. I like to think of meat as a condiment on the plate rather than the main event.

Meat adds flavor and texture, and it's a great source of protein. It's also the best delivery system for iron and vitamin B_{12}, and it contains other nutrients that can be more challenging to get in appreciable amounts from plant sources. So there are advantages to being an omnivore.

With that said, it's also important to consider the type and source of the meat you choose to eat. There's plenty of research to confirm that animals raised on their native diets in environments that are closer to their natural habitats will produce meat that is more nutrient-rich and less inflammatory. Assays on grass-fed beef confirm that there are more omega-3 fatty acids in their flesh than in that of grain-fed beef. The meats that are featured in this chapter were selected because they tend to be less inflammatory than other options. Lamb, for example, has a very unique fatty acid profile that mimics the ideal ratio of omega-6s to omega-3s for an anti-inflammatory diet.

My general words of wisdom for meat selection are:

» Look for 100 percent grass-fed beef and lamb (the labels "all natural" and even "organic" do not always mean 100 percent grass-fed)

» Take a walk on the wild side and try game meats or bison (buffalo)

» Choose free-range organic poultry

Moroccan Lamb Tagine with Chickpeas and Apricots

A traditional tagine would be made in an unusually shaped earthenware dish that resembles an upside down funnel. This version can be made right in your slow cooker. I recommend searing the meat and sautéing the onion the night before if you want to throw this together in the morning before work. Leave it to simmer while you're away and you'll be greeted by the mouthwatering aroma of a Moroccan-inspired mix of spices.

Makes 6 servings

¾ cup dried chickpeas, soaked overnight
2 teaspoons grapeseed oil
1 pound boneless lamb shoulder or leg, trimmed of fat and cut into 1-inch cubes
1 teaspoon sea salt, divided
Freshly ground black pepper
1 small yellow onion, diced
3½ cups beef broth

¾ cup dried apricots, chopped
5 cloves garlic, chopped
1 teaspoon minced peeled ginger
1 teaspoon ground turmeric
1 teaspoon ground cumin
½ teaspoon sweet paprika
½ teaspoon ground cinnamon
¼ teaspoon ground nutmeg
¼ cup chopped flat-leaf parsley

Rinse and drain the chickpeas and place in a slow cooker.

Heat the oil in a large skillet over medium-high heat. Add the lamb, season with ¼ teaspoon of the salt and pepper, and allow the pieces to brown on one side, 1 to 2 minutes. Turn the lamb pieces, season with another ¼ teaspoon of the salt and pepper, and allow the other sides to brown. Remove from the skillet with a slotted spoon and transfer to the slow cooker.

Add the onion to the skillet and sauté until it begins to brown. Transfer to the slow cooker.

Add the broth, apricots, garlic, ginger, turmeric, cumin, paprika, cinnamon, and nutmeg to the slow cooker and stir well. Cover and cook on low for 4 hours. Season with the remaining ½ teaspoon salt and stir in the parsley right before serving.

Bison Lettuce Cups with Garnet Yam Home Fries

Bison, or buffalo, is a naturally lean meat with a slightly stronger flavor than beef. Bison graze on their native diet of grass, so their meat is higher in omega-3s than red meat from animals that spend more time in the feedlots. I actually prefer the taste of bison to beef, and I think that sweet paprika, garlic, and pepper really elevate the savory flavors of the meat. Be sure to look for lettuce leaves that are large and somewhat pliable for best results. Or you can create dainty hors d'oeuvres using endive. The garnet yam fries are a universal hit and provide the perfect punch of color on the plate.

Makes 4 servings

2 unpeeled garnet yams, well scrubbed
2 teaspoons sunflower oil
1½ teaspoons coarse sea salt, divided
1 teaspoon five-spice powder
1 teaspoon coconut oil
1 pound ground bison (buffalo)
1 small white onion, chopped
2 carrots, shredded

1 yellow summer squash or zucchini, shredded
2 tablespoons chopped fresh oregano
2 teaspoons garlic powder
1 teaspoon sweet paprika
½ teaspoon freshly ground black pepper
½ teaspoon cayenne pepper
1 large head lettuce (I like Bibb or leaf lettuce)
¼ cup chopped green onions

Preheat the oven to 400 degrees F.

Cut the yams into strips the size of small steak fries (thinner if you prefer crispier fries). Toss with the sunflower oil, 1 teaspoon of the salt, and five-spice powder until well coated. Spread the fries evenly on a baking pan. Bake for 25 to 30 minutes, or until the fries start to brown and edges are becoming crispy. Turn off the oven, leaving the fries in there until ready to serve.

continued

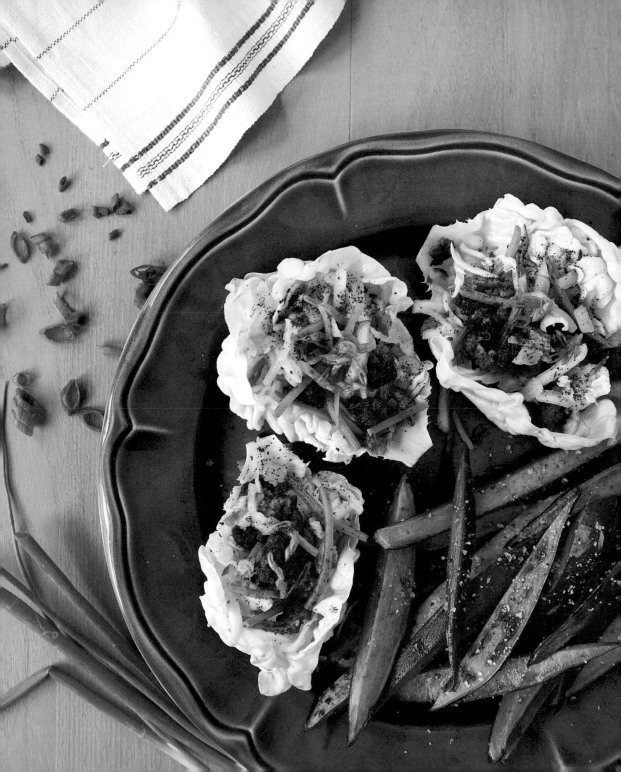

Heat the coconut oil in a large skillet over medium-high heat. Crumble the bison into the skillet and continue to break it up with a spatula as it cooks for 3 to 4 minutes. Use a slotted spoon to transfer the bison to a bowl. Add the onion and carrots to the skillet and sauté for 5 minutes. Add the squash and return the bison to the skillet. Stir in the oregano, garlic powder, paprika, remaining ½ teaspoon salt, pepper, and cayenne and sauté for 3 to 4 minutes.

To serve, scoop a generous helping of the bison mixture into a lettuce leaf and top with green onions. Repeat until you run out of filling or lettuce leaves. Place a couple lettuce cups on each plate and stack some yam fries beside them.

Tip: Use any leftover bison mixture as a topping on a green salad for a punch of flavor and boost of protein.

Spring Lamb Stew

This hearty stew is made lighter with fresh spring peas and mustard greens, and the flavors are spectacular! If parsnips are difficult to find, you can substitute sweet potatoes or regular potatoes if you're not avoiding nightshades. Lamb is an extremely healthy meat that has a better omega-6 to omega-3 ratio than most red meat, so it fits well into an anti-inflammatory diet. This stew could also be made in a slow cooker: just cook on low for six hours and add the kale thirty minutes before serving.

Makes 6 servings

1 tablespoon sunflower oil
2 pounds boneless lamb shoulder or
    leg, trimmed of fat and cut into
    1-inch cubes
Sea salt and freshly ground black
    pepper
1 yellow onion, chopped
6 large carrots, cut into 1-inch chunks
6 parsnips, cut into 1-inch chunks

3 cloves garlic, minced
½ cup dry white wine
2 teaspoons Dijon mustard
1 quart mushroom broth
2 cups chopped mustard greens
    or kale
1 cup fresh or frozen peas
1 cup chopped fresh parsley

Preheat the oven to 325 degrees F.

Heat the oil in large, deep cast-iron skillet or Dutch oven. Season the lamb to taste with salt and pepper. Add the lamb to the pan in a single layer and brown the meat on all sides. Use a slotted spoon to transfer the lamb to a bowl.

Add the onion to the pan and sauté until it begins to caramelize. Add the carrots, parsnips, and garlic and sauté for 5 minutes. Stir in the wine, mustard, and broth. Return the lamb to the pan and place it in the oven. Cook, uncovered, for about 1 hour, adding water as needed.

Stir in the greens, peas, and parsley and return the pan to the oven to cook for 15 to 20 minutes. Season to taste with salt and pepper and serve.

Steak Salad with Massaged Kale

This is a pretty interesting twist on steak salad and a great example of allowing vegetables to take center stage while the meat makes a flavorful cameo appearance. If you're just not sure about eating raw kale, do yourself a favor and try the massaged version. Playing rough with the kale helps break down the fibers and definitely makes it more enjoyable to eat raw. It also helps when the kale is marinating in a balsamic vinaigrette that's made creamy by our good friend Avocado. You can practice teamwork in the kitchen with your significant other if one of you loves to grill and the other prefers to manhandle the veggies.

Makes 4 servings

1 pound grass-fed flank or flatiron
   steak
2½ teaspoons coarse sea salt, divided
1 teaspoon dried Italian herbs
½ teaspoon freshly ground black
   pepper
¼ teaspoon freshly grated lemon zest

2 bunches Tuscan (Dino) kale,
   stemmed and roughly chopped
1 avocado
3 tablespoons balsamic vinegar
2 tablespoons extra-virgin olive oil
2 tablespoons agave nectar
2 carrots, shredded

Preheat a gas or charcoal grill.

Lay the steak out on a cutting board or baking pan. In a small bowl, combine 1 teaspoon of the salt, Italian herb blend, pepper, and lemon zest. Rub each side of the steak with the seasoning mixture.

Grill the steak over direct high heat for 4 minutes per side for medium-rare. Transfer to a plate, cover with foil, and allow the steak to rest for 5 minutes.

Meanwhile, put the kale in a large bowl. Scoop the avocado into the bowl. Drizzle in the balsamic vinegar, olive oil, agave, and remaining 1½ teaspoons salt. Using both hands, massage the avocado and dressing into the kale. It will start to take on a wilted appearance as it gets tender. Add the carrots and toss well.

Cut the steak across the grain into thin strips. Place a mound of salad on each plate and top with 4 or 5 steak strips.

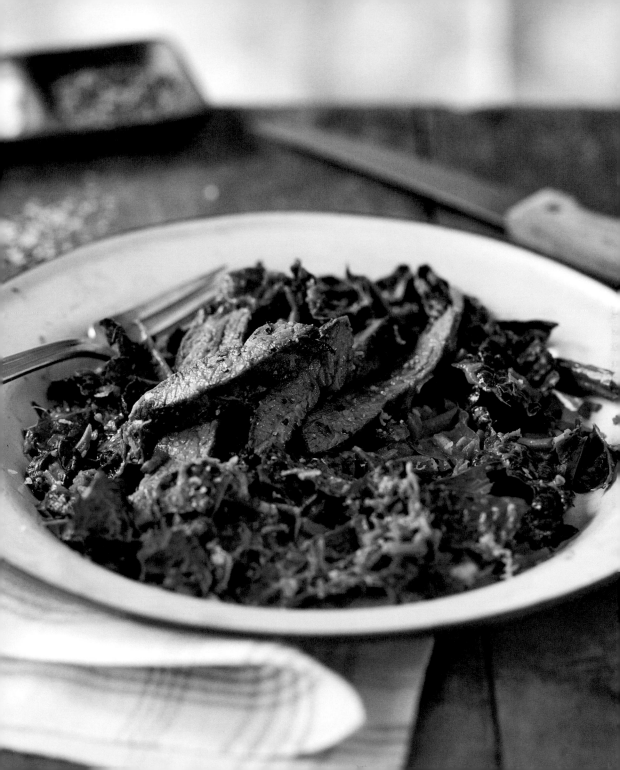

Veggie Beef Burger with Rocket Salad

I'm a sucker for a good, juicy burger, and I absolutely love the idea of embellishing it with some sautéed veggies mixed right into the meat. This whole concept was inspired by my turkey meatloaf, which gets its moisture from an array of vegetables that are discretely integrated. I discovered this translates well to beef burgers, and it's a good example of how to enjoy a bit of meat with a lot of veggies and still feel like you're eating a hearty, all-American meal. Rocket salad is the more descriptive British name for arugula. Although it's an adaptation of *roquette*, the French name for arugula, I like to think of it instead as a nod to the peppery flavor that blasts off in your mouth after the first bite.

Makes 4 servings

1 tablespoon sunflower oil
1 small yellow onion, diced
1 cup diced cremini mushrooms
1½ teaspoons sea salt, divided
1 carrot, shredded
1 small zucchini, shredded
1 pound ground grass-fed beef
¼ cup sunflower seeds
2 tablespoons dried parsley
2 teaspoons dried tarragon
1 teaspoon dried sage
½ teaspoon freshly ground
  black pepper

4 gluten-free hamburger buns
  (optional)

FOR THE SALAD:
2 tablespoons extra-virgin olive oil
1 tablespoon white balsamic vinegar
1 teaspoon stone-ground mustard
1 teaspoon honey
½ teaspoon sea salt
3 cups arugula
1 cup shredded purple cabbage
1 apple, cored and diced
1 English cucumber, chopped

To make the burgers, heat the sunflower oil in a large skillet or sauté pan over medium heat. Add the onion and sauté until it starts to become translucent. Add the mushrooms and 1 teaspoon of the salt and sauté for 5 minutes, or until the mushrooms start to release liquid and become soft. Add the carrot and zucchini and sauté for 2 to 3 minutes. Remove the skillet from the heat and let cool for 10 minutes.

Preheat a gas or charcoal grill.

Place the beef in a large mixing bowl. Add the sautéed vegetables, sunflower seeds, parsley, tarragon, sage, remaining ½ teaspoon salt, and pepper. Use both hands to knead the ingredients together until well combined. Form the mixture into 4 patties approximately ¾-inch thick.

Grill the patties over direct high heat for 8 to 10 minutes, turning once. Transfer to a plate, cover with foil, and allow the burgers to rest for 2 minutes.

To make the salad, whisk together the olive oil, vinegar, mustard, honey, and salt in a small bowl. Combine the arugula, cabbage, apple, and cucumber in a large bowl. Drizzle the vinaigrette over the salad and toss well to coat.

Place the burgers and a generous helping of salad on the gluten-free buns, or go bun-free and serve the salad in bowls with the burgers on top.

> Arugula is a great source of folic acid and rich in immune-boosting vitamins like A, C, and K. It's also a good plant-based source of calcium.

Sweet Potato Shepherd's Pie

Shepherd's pie is my rainy day, stay-in-my-PJs-and-watch-movies supper. This version of a classic comfort food foregoes the cream but features high-quality meat and a garlicky sweet potato topping. Even though this pie is made mostly from vegetables and is dotted with green peas, I still feel compelled to serve some greens on the side, like the Wilted Kale Salad with Shredded Beets and Carrots (page 93) or just some simple sautéed broccoli.

Makes 8 servings

1 head garlic
½ teaspoon extra-virgin olive oil
2 pounds sweet potatoes, peeled and cut into 1-inch cubes
¾ cup vegetable broth
1 pound ground bison, lamb, or grass-fed beef
1 teaspoon sea salt, plus more for seasoning

½ teaspoon freshly ground black pepper, plus more for seasoning
½ teaspoon ground nutmeg
1 small yellow onion, chopped
1 cup chopped cremini mushrooms
4 carrots, finely chopped
1 cup frozen peas

Preheat the oven to 400 degrees F.

Slice the top off the head of garlic to expose the cloves. Drizzle with the olive oil and wrap the head in foil. Place in the oven and roast for 50 minutes.

Meanwhile, place a steamer basket in a large saucepan with 1 inch of water. Put the sweet potatoes in the basket, cover the pan tightly, and steam for 15 to 20 minutes, or until the potatoes are tender and pierce easily with a fork. Drain and transfer the potatoes to the bowl of a food processor or stand mixer. Carefully squeeze the garlic cloves into the bowl. Add the broth and blend until the potatoes are thick and creamy. Season to taste with salt and pepper.

Turn on the broiler.

Place the bison in a large skillet over medium heat. Add the salt, pepper, and nutmeg and sauté the meat until brown. Use a slotted spoon to transfer the bison to a bowl.

Add the onion to the skillet and sauté until tender. Add the mushrooms and carrots, along with a little olive oil if needed, and sauté for 3 to 4 minutes. Add the peas and return the meat to the skillet. Cover and cook for 5 minutes.

Transfer the meat mixture to a 9-by-12-inch baking dish or deep pie pan and spread the sweet potatoes evenly over the top and to the edge of the pan. Place the dish in the oven and broil until the sweet potatoes begin to brown, 5 to 7 minutes.

> Sweet potatoes, which are not a member of the nightshade family, are an excellent source of complex carbohydrates and fiber.

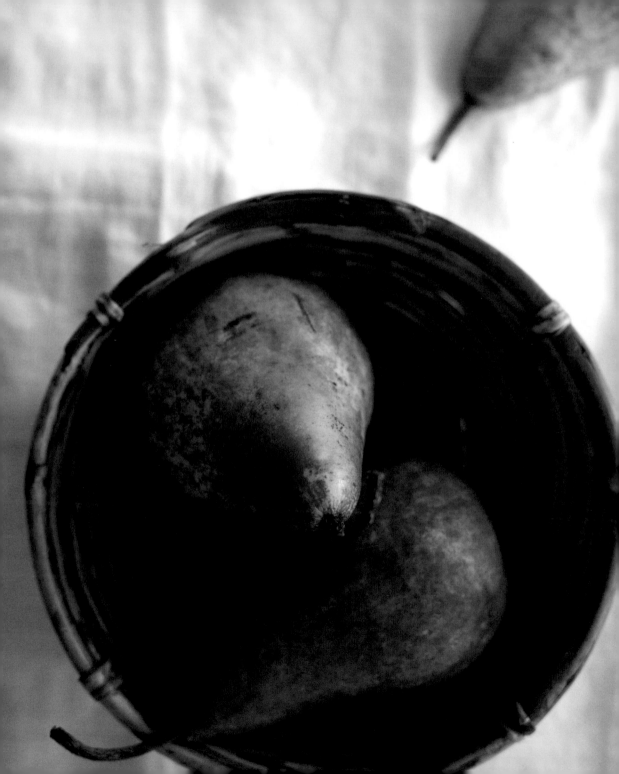

Desserts

Following an anti-inflammatory diet doesn't mean you don't get to have any treats. While refined sugar is high on the list of pro-inflammatory foods, there are plenty of great alternatives to satisfy a sweet tooth. Nature provides us with the best variety of desserts available in the form of fruits.

Sugar addicts may be rolling their eyes right now, doubting whether an apple could ever take the place of a chocolate frosted cupcake. The key is to get creative and learn what combinations of naturally decadent foods bring the same satisfaction and a lot less guilt (and pain!). Over time, your palate will even adjust to a lower level of sweetness, and fruits like mangoes and figs will give you as much of a sugar rush as you can handle.

In this chapter, you'll discover winning dessert combinations—like cashews and coconuts, dates and pecans—as well as lots of imaginative ways to use fruit. There's no chocolate on the menu, but that's only to make these recipes suitable for anyone on the anti-inflammatory cleanse; it's not explicitly forbidden otherwise. Cocoa is loaded with antioxidants and can also be used to create some amazing desserts. In fact, sometimes all you really need is a nice piece of dark chocolate.

Pumpkin Coconut Pie with Almond Crust

This pie is gluten-free, dairy-free, and absolutely delicious! Combining mildly sweet pumpkin with thick, rich coconut milk makes for a decadent filling that's sure to impress your dairy-loving friends. And since the crust is made from almonds and the filling is made from a vegetable in the squash family, it's a low-glycemic, guilt-free dessert. This recipe makes a double crust, but you'll only need half for a single pie, so the second portion can be frozen for up to three months for future use.

Makes 8 servings

FOR THE CRUST:
2 cups almond meal
⅓ cup arrowroot powder
1 teaspoon baking powder
1 teaspoon sea salt
½ teaspoon xanthan gum
⅓ cup coconut oil
¼ cup cold water

⸻⸻≫≫❯❮≪≪⸻

⅓ cup hot water
2 tablespoons ground flaxseed
2 cups pumpkin puree (canned is OK)
1 cup coconut milk
½ cup agave nectar or maple syrup
1 teaspoon ground cinnamon
1 teaspoon ground ginger
½ teaspoon sea salt
½ teaspoon freshly grated or ground nutmeg
¼ teaspoon ground cloves or allspice

To make the crust, in a large bowl, combine the almond meal, arrowroot powder, baking powder, salt, and xanthan gum and mix well. Add the coconut oil and blend with a fork or pastry cutter until the mixture is crumbly. Slowly stir in the water until the dough forms a ball. Divide into 2 equal balls, wrap in plastic wrap, and refrigerate for about 1 hour.

Preheat the oven to 375 degrees F.

continued

To make the filling, in a small bowl, stir together the hot water and flaxseed. Allow the mixture to sit for 10 minutes, then transfer to a large bowl. Add the pumpkin puree, coconut milk, agave, cinnamon, ginger, salt, nutmeg, and cloves and mix thoroughly.

Place 1 dough ball between 2 sheets of waxed paper and gently roll it out to about 10 inches in diameter. (The dough tears easily.) Carefully transfer the dough to a 9-inch pie pan and press it gently in place. Bake for 8 to 10 minutes to warm the crust. The crust may start to brown slightly. Pour the filling into the crust and bake for 35 to 45 minutes, or until the filling no longer jiggles. You may need to place foil around the edges if the crust starts to brown too much.

Let the pie cool completely and refrigerate for 2 to 3 hours before serving.

Tip: If you're not avoiding eggs, you can substitute 2 eggs in place of the hot water and flaxseed mixture.

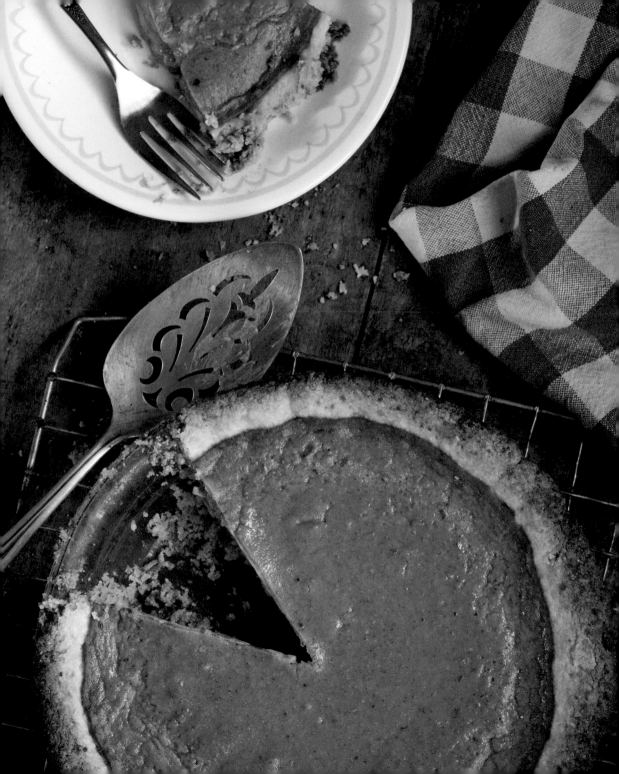

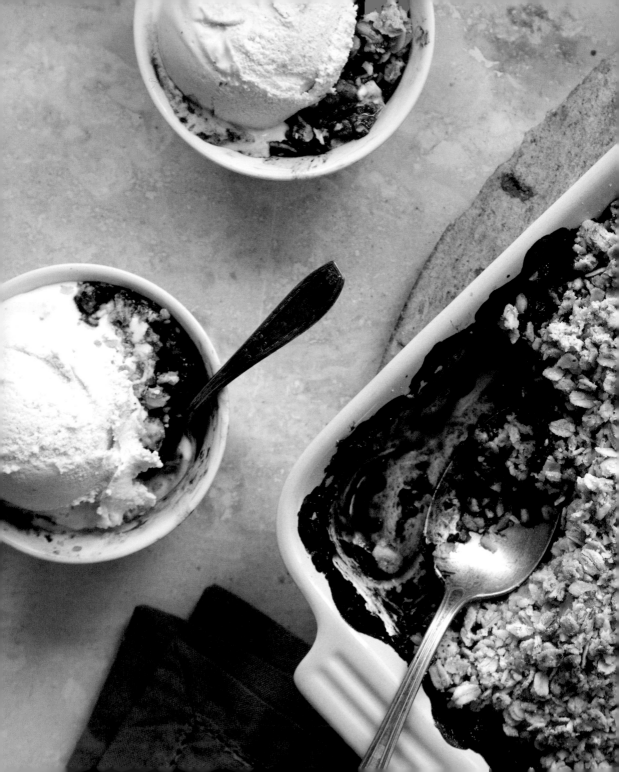

Mixed Berry Walnut Crumble

I love to make this dessert when my family comes to visit because everyone likes it, and it can double as breakfast the next morning. Trust me, no one ever complains about eating dessert for breakfast. When I'm serving it for dessert, I like to serve it warm and top it with some Coconut Bliss, a delicious nondairy ice cream substitute.

Makes 10 servings

FOR THE FILLING:
8 cups fresh or frozen mixed berries
¼ cup agave nectar
2 tablespoons arrowroot powder
1 teaspoon ground cinnamon
½ teaspoon ground nutmeg

2 cups certified gluten-free oats
1 cup chopped walnuts
½ cup brown rice flour
⅓ cup agave nectar
2 teaspoons ground cinnamon
½ teaspoon ground allspice
½ cup coconut oil, plus more for greasing dish

Preheat the oven to 350 degrees F. Lightly grease a 9-by-13-inch baking dish with coconut oil.

To make the filling, in a large bowl, combine the berries, agave, arrowroot powder, cinnamon, and nutmeg and toss until the berries are well coated. Transfer to the baking dish, cover with foil, and bake for 35 minutes.

Meanwhile, to make the topping, combine the oats, walnuts, flour, agave, cinnamon, and allspice in a medium bowl. Add the coconut oil and blend with a fork or pastry cutter until the mixture is crumbly.

Spread the topping over the fruit filling. Bake, uncovered, for 20 minutes, or until the topping is browned. Allow the crumble to cool slightly before serving.

Rustic Pear and Fig Crostatas

When I prepare this dessert in the cooking classes I teach, I tell students that the beauty of making a "rustic" dessert means that the crust doesn't have to look picture perfect. The amazingly easy gluten-free crust was inspired by a local gluten-free bakery called Flying Apron, and it can be a bit crumbly but it still works extremely well as a rustic wrap for fruit. The rich flavor of the figs blends beautifully with several varieties of pears, including Bartlett, Bosc, and Comice. This is sure to be a hit at any dinner party. Top it with cashew cream or some vanilla Coconut Bliss nondairy frozen dessert and you will think you've died and gone to heaven.

Makes 6 servings

7 to 8 fresh figs, cut into ½-inch chunks
1 large unpeeled pear, thinly sliced
1½ cups brown rice flour, plus more for dusting
¼ teaspoon sea salt

½ cup plus 3 tablespoons coconut oil
3 tablespoons agave nectar or maple syrup
1 to 2 tablespoons cold water
¼ cup honey

Preheat the oven to 350 degrees F.

Combine the figs and pear in a medium bowl and set aside.

In a small bowl, combine the flour and salt. In the bowl of a stand mixer fitted with the paddle attachment, beat the coconut oil until softened, about 1 minute. With the mixer on low speed, slowly add the flour mixture until incorporated. Add the agave and cold water and continue beating until a soft dough has formed. (Alternatively, you can mix the dough by hand, kneading the ingredients to incorporate.)

Dust a large piece of parchment paper (placed on top of a cutting board for ease) and your hands well with brown rice flour. Divide the dough into 6 equal balls. Flatten 1 ball and sprinkle with more flour. Roll the dough into a 4-inch disk. Spread 2 large spoonfuls of the fruit mixture into the center, leaving ½-inch of dough around the edges. Pull the dough up around the edges of the fruit, leaving the very center exposed. Repeat with the remaining dough balls and fruit.

Carefully transfer the parchment with the crostatas to a baking pan. Drizzle honey over the top of each crostata and bake for 25 minutes, or until the crusts are golden brown and the pears are soft.

Pears contain some unique phytonutrients called flavonols, which help improve blood sugar balance, support the immune system, and decrease inflammation.

So-Easy Coconut Mango Sorbet

Rich, creamy coconut milk and naturally sweet mangoes make this dessert seem absolutely sinful—but it's not! You can enjoy this quick and easy treat without a care in the world. For my clients who complain of having uncontrollable ice cream cravings when family members are enjoying theirs in front of them, this sorbet does the trick. You can experiment with different types of fruit, but there's something about the tropical combination of mangoes and coconut milk that provides just the right amount of sweetness and the perfect silky texture.

Makes 4 servings

1 (10-ounce) bag frozen mangoes
1 cup coconut milk

½ cup hazelnut or almond milk
½ teaspoon vanilla extract

Place all the ingredients in food processor or blender and blend until smooth. Serve immediately or freeze until the sorbet is the desired consistency.

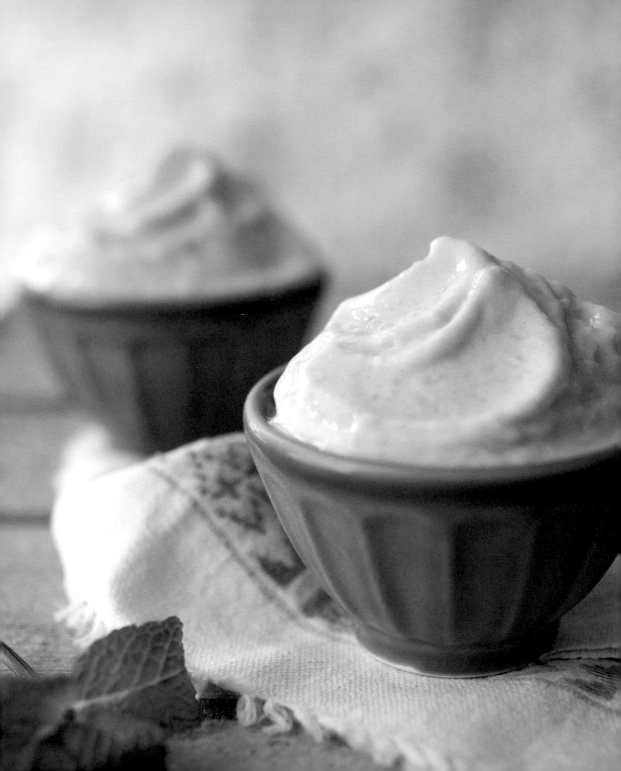

Baked Pears or Apples with Cashew Cream

Whenever I make cashew cream, I marvel at the simplicity of it! It's such a naturally delicious topping, and it pairs extremely well with baked pears or apples. Your house will smell like a freshly baked pie, and you'll have a healthy, satisfying dessert! The cashew cream is also great as a dip for raw fruit.

Makes 6 servings

3 large unpeeled pears or apples,
cored and halved
¾ cup water, divided

1 to 2 tablespoons ground cinnamon
2 tablespoons agave nectar
1 cup raw cashews

Preheat the oven to 375 degrees F.

Place the pears or apples face down in a medium baking dish. Add ½ cup of the water to the dish, cover with foil, and bake for 45 minutes. Uncover, sprinkle the fruit with cinnamon, drizzle with agave, and bake for another 5 minutes, or until the fruit is soft but not mushy.

Meanwhile, place the cashews in a food processor. With the machine running, slowly drizzle in the remaining ¼ cup water until the cream is the desired consistency.

Scoop the fruit into bowls and top with a heaping spoonful of cashew cream. Serve warm.

Strawberry Rhubarb Crumble

Strawberry rhubarb pie is definitely the way to my husband's heart. It reminds him of spending time in the kitchen with Grandma Babb on the farm. So I knew this recipe was a winner when my strawberry-rhubarb-pie connoisseur gave it the seal of approval and went back for seconds . . . and thirds. It doesn't last long in our house, but that's exactly what I expect of a good dessert.

Makes 8 servings

FOR THE FILLING:
⅓ cup coconut palm sugar
1½ tablespoons arrowroot powder
⅛ teaspoon sea salt
1 pound trimmed rhubarb, cut into
    ¼-inch-thick pieces (about 4 cups)
3 cups strawberries, hulled and
    quartered

——»»»≫≪«««——

½ cup coconut palm sugar
½ cup coconut flour
¼ cup white rice flour
1 teaspoon baking powder
½ teaspoon ground cinnamon
¼ teaspoon sea salt
½ cup certified gluten-free rolled oats
3 tablespoons hot water
1 tablespoon ground flaxseed
2 tablespoons agave nectar or
    maple syrup
¼ cup coconut oil, melted

Preheat the oven to 375 degrees F.

To make the filling, in a medium bowl, combine the coconut palm sugar, arrowroot powder, and salt. Add the rhubarb and strawberries, and gently toss until coated. Spread the fruit in a 10-inch pie pan and set aside.

To make the topping, in another medium bowl, combine the coconut palm sugar, flours, baking powder, cinnamon, and salt. Stir in the oats.

continued

In a small bowl, stir together the hot water and flaxseed. Allow the mixture to sit for 10 minutes, then add it to the dry ingredients. Stir in the agave. Using your hands, knead the ingredients until well combined. Sprinkle the topping evenly over the fruit. Drizzle the coconut oil evenly all over the topping.

Bake the crumble for 45 to 50 minutes, or until the topping turns a golden-brown color and the fruit is bubbling. Allow to cool slightly before serving.

Rhubarb is a good source of powerful antioxidants like lutein and lycopene, so it helps rid the body of free radicals that can cause inflammation and it keeps the immune system in check.

Vanilla Wafer Pudding

This recipe was a happy accident. I was trying to make macadamia nut cream, thinking it would have similar properties to cashew cream. Turns out that's not the case, but I kept adding ingredients to smooth out the texture and then put it the refrigerator and forgot about until the next day. When I pulled it out and had a couple bites, I kept feeling like it reminded me of something very familiar. A couple more bites and it dawned on me . . . it tastes exactly like vanilla wafers!

Makes 2 servings

1 cup raw macadamia nuts
½ ripe banana
¾ cup water

¼ cup coconut milk
2 teaspoons chia seeds
1 tablespoon agave nectar

Place all the ingredients in a food processor and blend until smooth. Transfer to an airtight container and refrigerate for at least 2 hours or overnight.

No-Bake Peach Pie

As a person who enjoys cooking much more than baking, there are a few qualities that make some desserts more desirable than others for me and this dessert has them all. It's simple, doesn't require baking, and it's absolutely decadent! I've made this pie using a variety of fruits, including mangoes, mixed berries, pears, and even fresh figs. You can't go wrong topping it with whatever is in season. Be sure to cut thin slices because the coconut cashew cream is extraordinarily rich and filling.

Makes 10 to 12 servings

FOR THE CRUST:
3 cups raw walnuts
¾ cup pitted dates (I prefer Medjool dates)
1 tablespoon ground cinnamon
¼ teaspoon sea salt

¾ cup hot water
½ cup creamed coconut, chopped into chunks
2 cups raw cashews
2 tablespoons maple syrup
Seeds from 1 vanilla bean
3 ripe peaches, peeled and thinly sliced

To make the crust, combine the walnuts, dates, cinnamon, and salt in a food processor and blend until the ingredients are finely chopped and well combined.

Scrape the mixture into a 9-inch pie pan greased with coconut oil. Press into the bottom of the pan, pushing the crust up to reach the top edge all around. Wash the food processor before proceeding.

To make the filling, put the hot water and creamed coconut in the food processor and let sit for 5 minutes so the coconut can soften. Add the cashews, maple syrup, and vanilla bean seeds and blend until smooth.

Spread the cream evenly into the crust. Arrange the peaches in a circular pattern over the cream filling. Can be served immediately.

> Walnuts contain higher amounts of omega-3s than any other nut and are a rich source of unique anti-inflammatory phytonutrients.

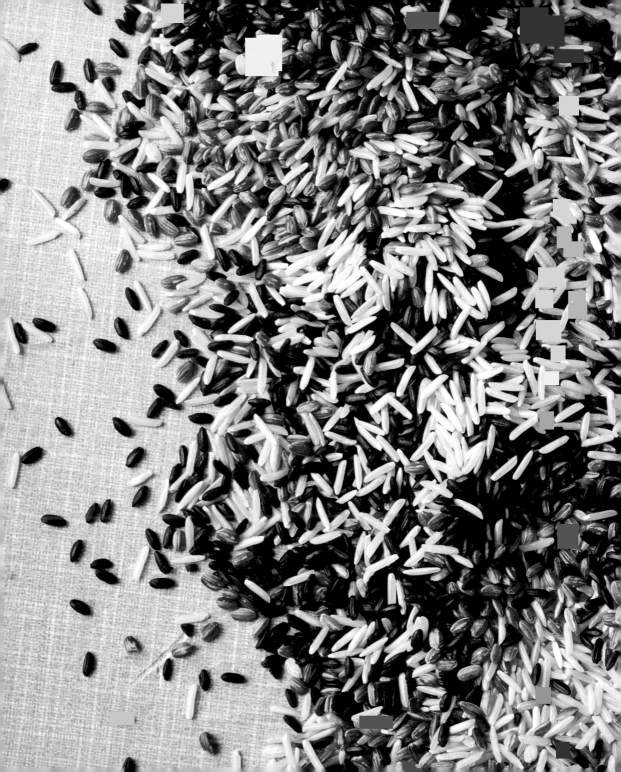

Acknowledgments

It takes a village to write a cookbook, and I couldn't have done it without the constant encouragement and support from my incredibly patient husband along with my family, friends, and colleagues. Barb Schiltz put me on the path to becoming a nutritionist and I will be forever indebted to her for helping me find my true passion. She's my mentor, sage (in the non-herbal sense), and favorite cooking companion.

I developed my love for cooking later in life, when I was a grad student at Bastyr University. I took my first whole foods cooking class from Cynthia Lair and I was hooked. She made healthy cooking accessible and exciting and she didn't even ridicule me when I showed up on the first day with an herb knife instead of a chef's knife.

Four years later, I was developing and teaching my own cooking classes with a nutritional bent. I will be infinitely grateful to the incredibly organized team at Puget Consumers Co-op (PCC), Marilyn McCormick, Jackie DeCicco, and Alicia Guy, to name a few. It's because of them that the anti-inflammatory cooking classes I teach get noticed and are well attended. I'm proud to be a part of a co-op that can boast being one of the largest cooking schools in the nation.

The recipes in this book are a labor of love and a reflection of my passion. They also went through several rounds of tasting and tweaking. Heartfelt gratitude to my fabulous recipe testers, Bill Babb, Maribeth Evezich, Kim Campbell, Jenny Harris, Rob Sweet, and Vicki Duffy. You've made these delicious dishes infinitely better with your thoughtful comments and food-savvy suggestions. And a big thank you to my mom, who didn't make the cut for recipe tester because of her mysterious aversion to all herbs and spices, but she's always there to cheer me on and celebrate my successes.

Now let's eat!

Index

Conversions

VOLUME

US	METRIC	IMPERIAL
¼ tsp.	1.25 ml	
½ tsp.	2.5 ml	
1 tsp.	5 ml	
½ Tbsp.	7.5 ml	
1 Tbsp.	15 ml	
⅛ c.	30 ml	1 fl. oz.
¼ c.	60 ml	2 fl. oz.
⅓ c.	80 ml	2.5 fl. oz.
½ c.	125 ml	4 fl. oz.
1 c.	250 ml	8 fl. oz.
2 c. (1 pt.)	500 ml	16 fl. oz.
1 qt.	1 l	32 fl. oz.

LENGTH

US	METRIC
⅛ in.	3 mm
¼ in.	6 mm
½ in.	1.25 cm
1 in.	2.5 cm
1 ft.	30 cm

WEIGHT

AVOIRDUPOIS	METRIC
¼ oz.	7 g
½ oz.	15 g
1 oz.	30 g
2 oz.	60 g
3 oz.	90 g
4 oz.	115 g
5 oz.	150 g
6 oz.	175 g
7 oz.	200 g
8 oz. (½ lb.)	225 g
9 oz.	250 g
10 oz.	300 g
11 oz.	325 g
12 oz.	350 g
13 oz.	375 g
14 oz.	400 g
15 oz.	425 g
16 oz. (1 lb.)	450 g
1½ lb.	750 g
2 lb.	900 g
2¼ lb.	1 kg
3 lb.	1.4 kg
4 lb.	1.8 kg

TEMPERATURE

OVEN MARK	FAHRENHEIT	CELSIUS	GAS
Very cool	250–275	130–140	½–1
Cool	300	150	2
Warm	325	165	3
Moderate	350	175	4
Moderately hot	375	190	5
	400	200	6
Hot	425	220	7
	450	230	8
Very Hot	475	245	9

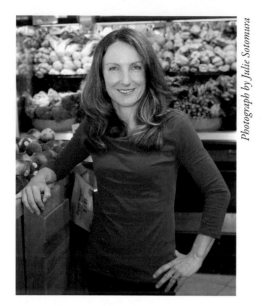

Photograph by Julie Sotomura

About the Author

MICHELLE BABB is a registered dietitian with a private practice in West Seattle, where she specializes in mind-body nutrition, weight management, and inflammatory digestive disorders.

Michelle developed a passion for cooking when she was a student at Bastyr, and now teaches nutrition-focused cooking classes at Puget Consumers Co-op. Her recipes often feature underappreciated ingredients, like beets, brussels sprouts, and Jerusalem artichokes. She takes great pleasure in converting dubious meat and potato lovers into vegetable enthusiasts.

When she's not in the kitchen, Michelle enjoys running, kayaking, sailing, and traveling. She also loves to write and is co-author of *The Imperfect Perfectionist: Seasonal Secrets for a Happy and Balanced Life*. Learn more about Michelle at EatPlayBe.com.